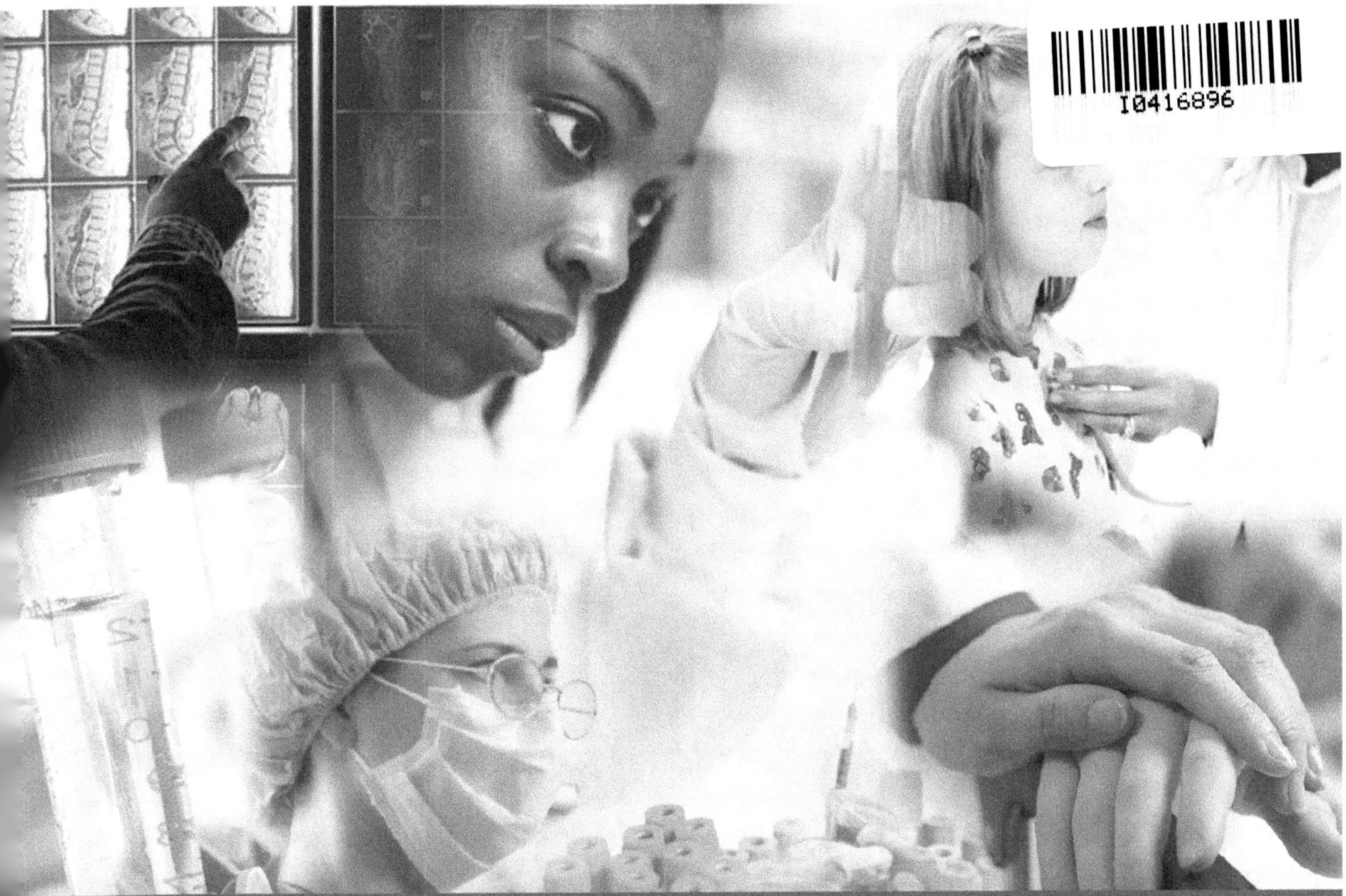

Healthcare and Public Health Sector-Specific Plan

An Annex to the National Infrastructure Protection Plan

2010

Homeland Security

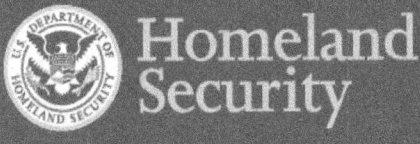

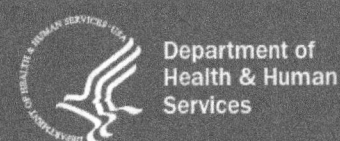

Department of Health & Human Services

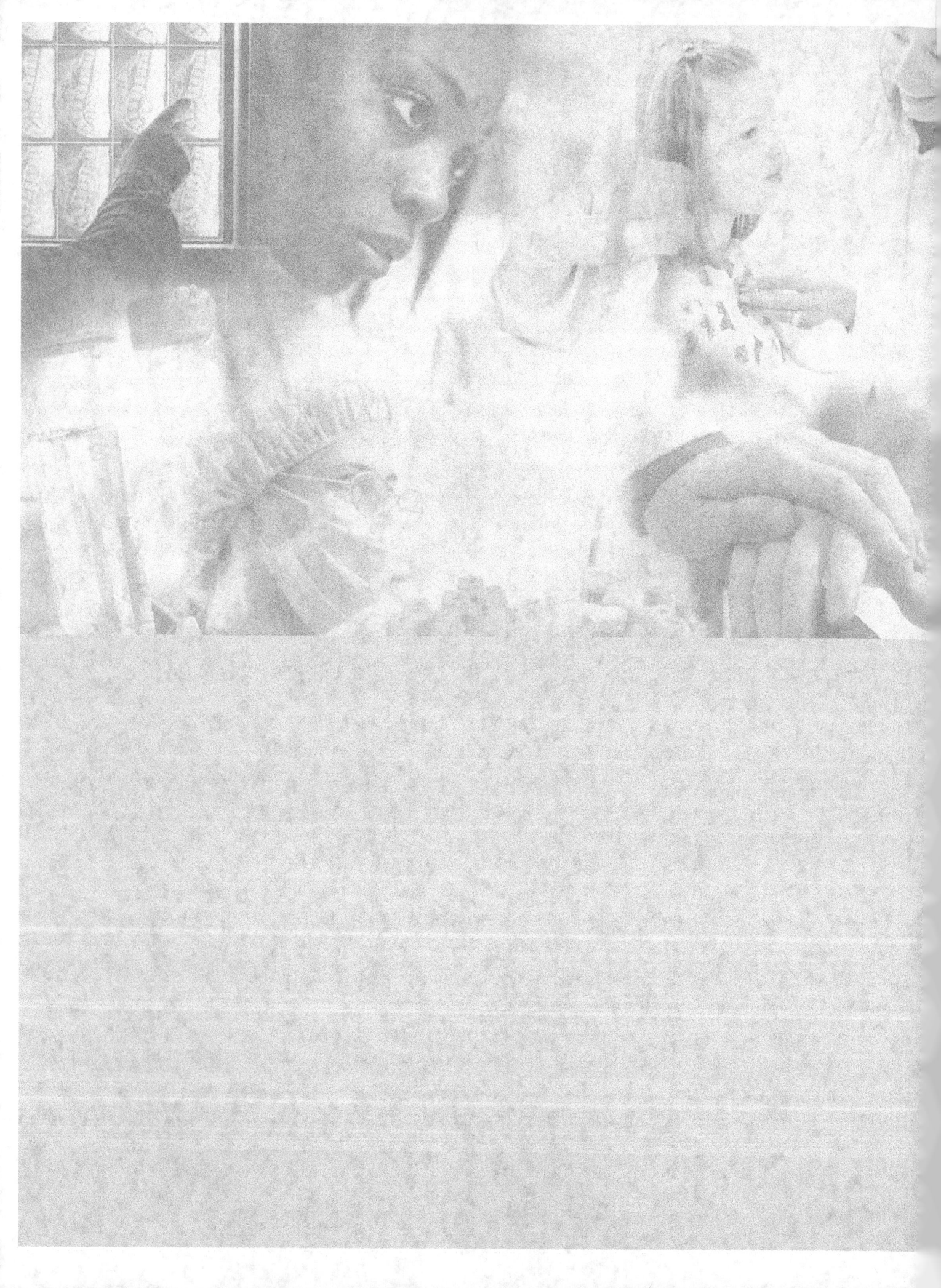

Preface

The Healthcare and Public Health (HPH) Sector constitutes a significant portion of the U.S. economy. The U.S. Department of Health and Human Services (HHS) estimates that 16.2% ($2.2 trillion) of our Nation's 2007 Gross Domestic Product (GDP) was spent on healthcare and this percentage was expected to increase to 17.6% in 2009. Privately owned and operated organizations comprise the vast majority of the sector and identify themselves with the delivery of healthcare goods and services. The public health component consists largely of government agencies at the Federal, State, local, tribal, and territorial levels. Due to the diffuse nature of the sector, there are many targets for potential attack that are exceptionally hard to protect. A breakdown in the healthcare infrastructure would result in a significant impact on the economy, a loss of human life, and a breakdown in other critical sectors. To help manage this risk, HHS and its government and private sector partners have developed this Healthcare and Public Health Sector-Specific Plan (HPH SSP).

This SSP provides the unifying structure for the integration of HPH protection efforts into a single national program to help achieve the goal of a safe, secure, and resilient America through enhanced protection of the Nation's critical infrastructure and key resources (CIKR). As an annex to the National Infrastructure Protection Plan (NIPP), the HPH SSP describes how the NIPP risk management framework is being implemented and integrated within the HPH Sector.

This 2010 release of the HPH SSP reflects the maturation of the Healthcare and Public Health Sector partnership and the progress of the sector programs first outlined in the 2007 SSP. Changes from the 2007 SSP include a streamlined and updated set of goals and objectives and an increased emphasis on priorities such as information sharing and emergency response. Examples of HPH accomplishments since the publication of the 2007 SSP include the following:

- The sector launched new programs and working groups to address sector challenges, including the Private Sector Liaison Officers Program, Cybersecurity Working Group, and Information Sharing Working Group.

- The Homeland Security Information Network HPH portal was expanded and re-launched to better meet the information-sharing needs of the sector.

- Both the Sector Coordinating Council and Government Coordinating Council undertook extensive outreach programs. State, local, and private sector partners were recruited through presentations, webinars, and outreach to national associations.

- The sector updated various approaches to disasters based on lessons from the H1N1 pandemic; hurricanes Gustav, Hannah, and Ike; and the Conficker worm.

- The number of Metropolitan Statistical Areas (MSAs) that meet Cities Readiness Initiative criteria for effectively distributing medical countermeasures increased by 30 percent.

- The number of security site audits at medical countermeasure facilities doubled.

The HPH Sector continues to take steps to better understand risks to the sector from all hazards. To address these risks, the sector is implementing risk mitigation activities (RMAs) at all levels of government and the private sector. RMAs described in this SSP include the following:

- Federal cooperative agreement programs such as the Public Health Emergency Preparedness Program, which builds State, territorial, and local health department resilience; and the Hospital Preparedness Program (HPP), which builds resilience at healthcare facilities;

- Federal regulatory programs such as the Select Agent Program, which oversees laboratories and other entities that possess, use, or transfer certain biological agents and toxins; and

- Voluntary private sector initiatives such as RxResponse and the sector's Medical Materials Coordinating Group, which work to enhance supply chain resilience for drugs, biological products, and medical devices.

Each year, the Healthcare and Public Health Sector CIKR Protection Annual Report will provide updates on the sector's efforts to identify, prioritize, and coordinate the protection of its critical infrastructure. The Sector Annual Report provides the current priorities of the sector as well as the progress made during the past year in following the plans and strategies set out in the HPH SSP.

This SSP represents a collaborative effort between the private sector; State, local, tribal, and territorial governments; nongovernmental organizations; and the Federal Government. This collaboration will result in the prioritization of protection initiatives and investments within and across sectors to deter threats, decrease vulnerabilities, and minimize the consequences of attacks and other incidents.

The Healthcare and Public Health Sector Coordinating Council and Government Coordinating Council are pleased to support this SSP and look forward to sustaining and enhancing the protection and resilience of critical infrastructure in the HPH Sector.

Nitin Natarajan

Chair, HPH Sector
Government Coordinating Council
U.S. Department of
Health and Human Services

Todd M. Keil

Assistant Secretary for
Infrastructure Protection
U.S. Department of
Homeland Security

Al Cook

Chief Resource Director
Regional Medical Center
Tri-Chair, HPH Sector
Coordinating Council

David Morgan

Owner/Operator
Brooklawn Memorial Park
Tri-Chair, HPH Sector
Coordinating Council

Erin Mullen, RPh, PhD

Assistant VP
Rx Response PhRMA
Tri-Chair, HPH Sector
Coordinating Council

Table of Contents

Preface i

Executive Summary 1

    1. Sector Profile and Goals 1

    2. Identify Assets, Systems, and Networks 2

    3. Assess Risks 2

    4. Prioritize Infrastructure 3

    5. Develop and Implement Protective Programs and Resilience Strategies 3

    6. Measure Effectiveness 4

    7. CIKR Protection Research and Development 4

    8. Managing and Coordinating Sector-Specific Agency Responsibilities 5

Introduction 7

1. Sector Profile and Goals 9

    1.1 Sector Profile 9

        1.1.1 Significant Dependencies 11

        1.1.2 Significant Overlaps 12

        1.1.3 Authorities Governing the Sector 12

    1.2 Sector Partners 13

        1.2.1 Coordinating Councils 13

        1.2.2 Department of Homeland Security 14

        1.2.3 Other Federal Partners 14

        1.2.4 Cross-Sector Groups and Regional Coalitions 15

    1.3 Sector Vision, Mission, Goals and Objectives 15

    1.4 Value Proposition 18

2. Identify Assets, Systems, and Networks 19

    2.1 Defining Information Parameters 19

    2.2 Collecting Infrastructure Information 20

    2.3 Verifying and Updating Infrastructure Information 21

    2.4 The Path Forward 21

3. Assess Risks **23**

    3.1 Use of Risk Assessment in the Sector. 23

    3.2 Assessing Vulnerabilities and Consequences 24

        3.2.1 Strategic Homeland Infrastructure Risk Analysis 24

        3.2.2 Network Analysis 24

        3.2.3 Healthcare Facility Risk and Design Analysis Tool 24

        3.2.4 Cybersecurity Risk Assessment. 25

    3.3 Path Forward. 26

4. Prioritize Infrastructure **27**

    4.1 Current Prioritization Process 27

    4.2 The Path Forward 27

5. Develop and Implement Protective Programs and Resilience Strategies **29**

    5.1 Overview of Sector Protective Programs and Resilience Strategies 29

    5.2 Determining the Need for Protective Programs and Resilience Strategies 31

    5.3 Protective Program/Resilience Strategy Implementation. 31

    5.4 Monitoring Program Implementation 31

    5.5 Path Forward. 32

6. Measure Effectiveness **33**

    6.1 Risk Mitigation Activities 33

    6.2 Process for Measuring Effectiveness 33

    6.3 Using Metrics for Continuous Improvement 34

    6.4 Path Forward. 34

7. CIKR Protection Research & Development **35**

    7.1 R&D Management Processes 35

    7.2 R&D Priorities and Capability Gaps. 36

    7.3 Path Forward. 37

8. Managing and Coordinating SSA Responsibilities **39**

    8.1 Program Management Approach. 39

    8.2 Processes and Responsibilities. 39

        8.2.1 SSP Maintenance and Update. 39

        8.2.2 Resources and Budgets. 39

        8.2.3 Training and Education. 40

    8.3 Implementing the Partnership Model 40

      8.3.1 NIPP Coordinating Structures 40

      8.3.2 Advisory Councils and Committees 41

      8.3.3 Academia, Research Centers, and Think Tanks 42

      8.3.4 International Organizations 42

   8.4 Information Sharing and Protection 42

   8.5 The Path Forward 43

   8.6 SSP Implementation Actions 43

Appendix 1: List of Acronyms and Abbreviations 45

Appendix 2: Authorities Governing the Sector 47

Appendix 3: Healthcare and Public Health Sector Coordinating Council Member Organizations 53

Appendix 4: Healthcare and Public Health Sector Government Coordinating Council Member Organizations 57

Appendix 5: Implementation Considerations for State, Local, Tribal, Territorial, and Private Sector Partners 59

List of Tables

Table 1-1:   Healthcare and Public Health Sector Statistics 11

Table 1-2:   Sector Dependencies 12

Table 1-3:   HPH Sector Goals 16

Table 1-4:   HPH Sector Objectives 17

Table 3-1:   Common Cyber Threats, Vulnerabilities, Consequences, and Mitigation Strategies 25

Table 7-1:   Sector R&D Priorities and Capability Gap Statements Mapped to Sector Goals and NIPP CIP R&D Themes 36

Table 8-1:   SSP Implementation Actions 43

Table A2-1: Summary of Major HPH Sector Federal Authorities by Agency and Function 47

List of Figures

Figure I-1: NIPP Risk Management Framework 7

Figure 1-1: HPH Sector Vision and Mission 16

Figure 2-2: The DHS Data Call Process 20

Figure 8-1: Sector Partnership Model 41

Executive Summary

The Healthcare and Public Health (HPH) Sector-Specific Plan (SSP) complements the National Infrastructure Protection Plan (NIPP) by detailing the application of the NIPP framework to the unique characteristics and risk landscape of the sector. The SSP lays out a collaborative process among government and private sector partners to protect the HPH Sector from natural disasters, pandemics, terrorist attacks, and other manmade disasters, referred to collectively as "all hazards." The plan describes current processes and sets a path forward for the sector to cooperatively identify and prioritize its assets, assess risk, implement protective programs, and measure the effectiveness of its protective programs. It summarizes research and development (R&D) activities in the sector and describes the sector's approach to managing its responsibilities in the areas of partnership, training and education, and information sharing and protection.

The SSP is divided into eight chapters, based on the NIPP risk management framework and other sector responsibilities. A brief summary of each chapter follows.

1. Sector Profile and Goals

Chapter 1 gives a profile of the sector and states the sector's vision, mission, and goals.

The HPH Sector is vast and diverse. The sector employs approximately 13 million personnel and represents an estimated 16.2 percent ($2.2 trillion) of our Nation's Gross Domestic Product (GDP). It includes not only acute care hospitals and ambulatory healthcare, but also the vast and complex public-private systems that finance that care. It includes population-based care provided by health agencies at the Federal, State, local, tribal, and territorial levels, as well as other public health and disease surveillance functions. It incorporates a large system of private sector enterprises that manufacture, distribute, and sell drugs, vaccines, and medical supplies and equipment, as well as a network of small businesses that provide mortuary services. All of these goods and services are provided in and by means of a complex environment of research, regulation, finance, and public policy.

Sector Vision

The HPH Sector will achieve overall resilience against all hazards. It will prevent or minimize damage to, or destruction of, the Nation's healthcare and public health infrastructure. It will strive to protect its workforce and preserve its ability to mount timely and effective responses (without disruption to services in unaffected areas) and to recover from both routine and emergency situations.

Sector Mission

The mission of the HPH Sector is to sustain the essential functions of the Nation's healthcare and public health delivery system and to support effective emergency preparedness and response to nationally significant hazards by implementing strategies, evaluating risks, coordinating plans and policy advice, and providing guidance to prepare, protect, prevent, and, when necessary, respond to attacks on the Nation's infrastructure, and support the necessary resilience in infrastructure to recover and reconstitute healthcare and public health services.

Sector Goals

The HPH Sector has established four goals in the areas of service continuity, workforce protection, physical asset protection, and cybersecurity:

- **Service Continuity**—Maintain the ability to provide essential health services during and after disasters or disruptions in the availability of supplies or supporting services (e.g., water, power);
- **Workforce Protection**—Protect the sector's workforce from the harmful consequences of all hazards that may compromise their health and safety and limit their ability to carry out their responsibilities;
- **Physical Asset Protection**—Mitigate the risks posed by all hazards to the sector's physical assets; and
- **Cybersecurity**—Mitigate risks to the sector's cyber assets that may result in disruption to or denial of health services.

2. Identify Assets, Systems, and Networks

Chapter 2 discusses the HPH Sector's processes for identifying critical assets, systems, and networks, and explains the infrastructure information collection methods that support sector critical infrastructure and key resources (CIKR) protection efforts.

The HPH Sector is developing a functional model that provides a framework for identifying assets, systems, and networks. With the model, the sector can evaluate functions and determine the underlying infrastructure necessary to support these functions. The functional model enables the sector to view its infrastructure from a business continuity perspective.

The HPH Sector participates in the National Critical Infrastructure Prioritization Program (NCIPP) led by the U.S. Department of Homeland Security (DHS). In support of this program, the HPH Sector develops and refines criteria for identifying HPH Sector critical assets. The sector partners with DHS to gather, validate, and prioritize the list of critical HPH assets that are of national significance.

Moving forward, the sector will continue defining the functions of the HPH Sector to support an analysis of the underlying infrastructure necessary to perform these functions. The sector will expand its involvement in NCIPP to identify an additional level of assets that do not meet the criteria for national significance, but which are critical at the sector and regional levels.

3. Assess Risks

Chapter 3 provides information on the HPH Sector's approach for assessing risk. It includes information on a selection of risk analysis tools and describes vulnerability and consequence assessment in the sector.

The risk analysis performed in the HPH Sector is conducted to achieve compliance with safety, physical security, and information security regulations. Beyond the need to meet regulatory requirements, HPH Sector organizations have a vested interest in conducting risk analysis to identify risks that could lead to negative financial consequences and damage to their reputations.

The sector is actively involved in several vulnerability and consequence assessment activities. The sector participates in the DHS Strategic Homeland Infrastructure Risk Analysis (SHIRA) process. SHIRA establishes a common framework by which sectors can assess the economic, loss of life, and psychological consequences resulting from all hazards. The sector is also using the functional model it is developing to conduct a network analysis that examines sector interdependencies, external dependencies, and critical nodes. The network analysis exposes underlying vulnerabilities and potential points of failure and enables the sector to analyze cascading consequences that result from the failure of a function and to develop risk management strategies. In addition to this work, the sector is developing a healthcare facility security and design analysis tool for use by building owners and designers to analyze the security risks of an organization based on geographic location, natural hazards, and service types to facilitate optimal design options for security and medical surge. The sector is also performing a cybersecurity risk assessment as part of its work in creating a sector cybersecurity strategy.

The sector will continue to build its risk assessment capability through the use of risk assessment tools and network analysis. The sector will evaluate available risk assessment tools and educate its members on their use. The sector will also continue to leverage the network analysis to inform its risk mitigation activities.

4. Prioritize Infrastructure

Chapter 4 discusses the sector's current process and path forward for prioritizing its critical assets, systems, and networks.

The HPH Sector's current prioritization process occurs through its participation in NCIPP. In partnership with the U.S. Department of Health and Human Services (HHS), DHS conducts a consequence-based risk assessment to determine which critical assets are of national significance and thus should be prioritized ahead of other sector assets.

Using the criteria it developed for NCIPP, the sector plans to expand its current prioritization process to include the formal identification of a third level of assets. Where prioritization at an asset, system, or network level is not possible, the sector will prioritize subsectors for specific threats.

5. Develop and Implement Protective Programs and Resilience Strategies

Chapter 5 describes some of the major projective programs in the sector and the current processes for identifying critical infrastructure protection (CIP) needs and implementing CIP programs.

Government and private sector organizations develop and implement protective programs and resilience strategies to address a wide range of challenges that relate to the sector's goals of service continuity, workforce protection, physical asset protection, and cybersecurity. HHS facilitates communication between government and private sector organizations to increase collaboration and the effectiveness of the sector's protective programs and resilience strategies. Detailed descriptions of significant protective programs and resilience initiatives are available in the HPH Sector Annual Report (SAR).

Legislative and regulatory mandates drive many of the government programs and resilience strategies in the HPH Sector. Congress identifies CIP needs and creates Federal programs and strategies to address these needs. State, local, tribal, and territorial governments also assess unique CIP needs in their jurisdictions and develop corresponding programs to address these needs. Many private sector organizations in the HPH Sector assess risks to their infrastructure as part of their business continuity programs.

Government and private sector organizations from across the HPH Sector implement protective programs and resilience strategies with varying degrees of coordination. The HPH Sector will continue to foster an environment where public and private sector organizations can communicate about their programs and collaborate when possible to achieve maximum effectiveness.

6. Measure Effectiveness

Chapter 6 describes the processes used by the sector to measure the effectiveness of its protective programs and use this information to continuously improve them.

The sector relies on performance measurement done at the program level to indicate progress toward achieving its CIP goals and objectives. Most federally funded programs require grant awardees to report their progress annually. The agencies that manage these programs provide this performance data for use in determining and reporting on CIP progress in the sector.

The sector also measures engagement in its CIP program. Metrics based on participation in CIP meetings, use of the sector's information-sharing portal, and participation in work groups provide meaningful information about the progress of the sector's CIP program.

Increasingly, Federal agencies that fund and administer large CIP-related programs base future funding decisions on the performance of grant awardees. At the macro level, Congress, the Office of Management and Budget, and other Federal oversight organizations review the effectiveness of large CIP-related programs, and may increase funding for effective programs and reduce or eliminate funding for ineffective programs.

Moving forward, the CIP Program Office will continue to partner with organizations that fund large CIP programs to leverage their performance management data and measure CIP program engagement. The program office will also work with these organizations to add measures to their performance management systems that are CIP-focused.

7. CIKR Protection Research and Development

Chapter 7 describes the sector's approach to managing its R&D activities and provides a list of the sector's current R&D priorities and capability gaps.

HPH Sector members devote significant time and resources to developing R&D and Modeling, Simulation, and Analysis (MS&A) requirements. The process includes an environmental scan of current and historical research to limit the potential for duplicative projects. The sector reviews its R&D and MS&A portfolio yearly to ascertain how best to dedicate time and resources and to review the status of the previous year's efforts. The sector develops capability gap statements to describe areas where additional research is needed to improve sector protection and resilience. Sector leadership maintains a high degree of visibility into the progress of these projects, reviewing requests for proposals, proposals, and deliverables from each of the initiatives.

The sector focuses its R&D efforts on developing requirements that improve its ability to manage medical surge and sustain its workforce and supply chain during an all-hazards incident. The sector recently added cyber infrastructure protection as an R&D priority. In 2009, the Joint Advisory Work Group (JAWG) submitted 17 capability gap statements in support of these priorities. The gap statements are available in the 2009 HPH SAR. Moving forward, the focus of the sector will shift from the development of new capability gap statements to the implementation and monitoring of research projects that address previously submitted capability gap statements.

8. Managing and Coordinating Sector-Specific Agency Responsibilities

Chapter 8 describes the management processes and partnership model that HHS has established to meet its responsibilities under Homeland Security Presidential Directive 7 (HSPD-7) and related guidance. It also describes the information-sharing mechanisms in use in the sector.

The Office of the Assistant Secretary for Preparedness and Response (ASPR) in HHS leads CIKR protection efforts for the HPH Sector. ASPR is responsible for developing and maintaining relationships with public and private sector partners. To do this, ASPR has established a Sector Coordinating Council (SCC), Government Coordinating Council (GCC), and several joint work groups under the auspices of the Critical Infrastructure Partnership Advisory Council (CIPAC). The SCC is a self-governing body representing the health industry that provides a forum for the private sector to discuss infrastructure protection issues and communicate with government. The GCC is the public sector component of the sector's public-private partnership framework; it includes representatives from across Federal, State, local, tribal, and territorial governments. Members from these two councils are brought together to serve on joint work groups pursuant to CIPAC.

The HPH Sector invests significant resources in initiatives to continually expand its information-sharing capabilities. These initiatives include the enhancement and rollout of the Homeland Security Information Network (HSIN) HPH portal and the implementation of notification and alert capabilities. In response to all-hazards events, the SSA initiates conference calls open to the entire sector to accelerate communications. These information-sharing initiatives deliver considerable value to sector members and have significantly increased engagement in the CIP program.

Moving forward, the sector will continue to make use of CIPAC to establish work groups focused on meeting its goals and objectives. The sector will also continue to expand its use of HSIN-HPH by identifying and posting additional information products and increasing the number of users.

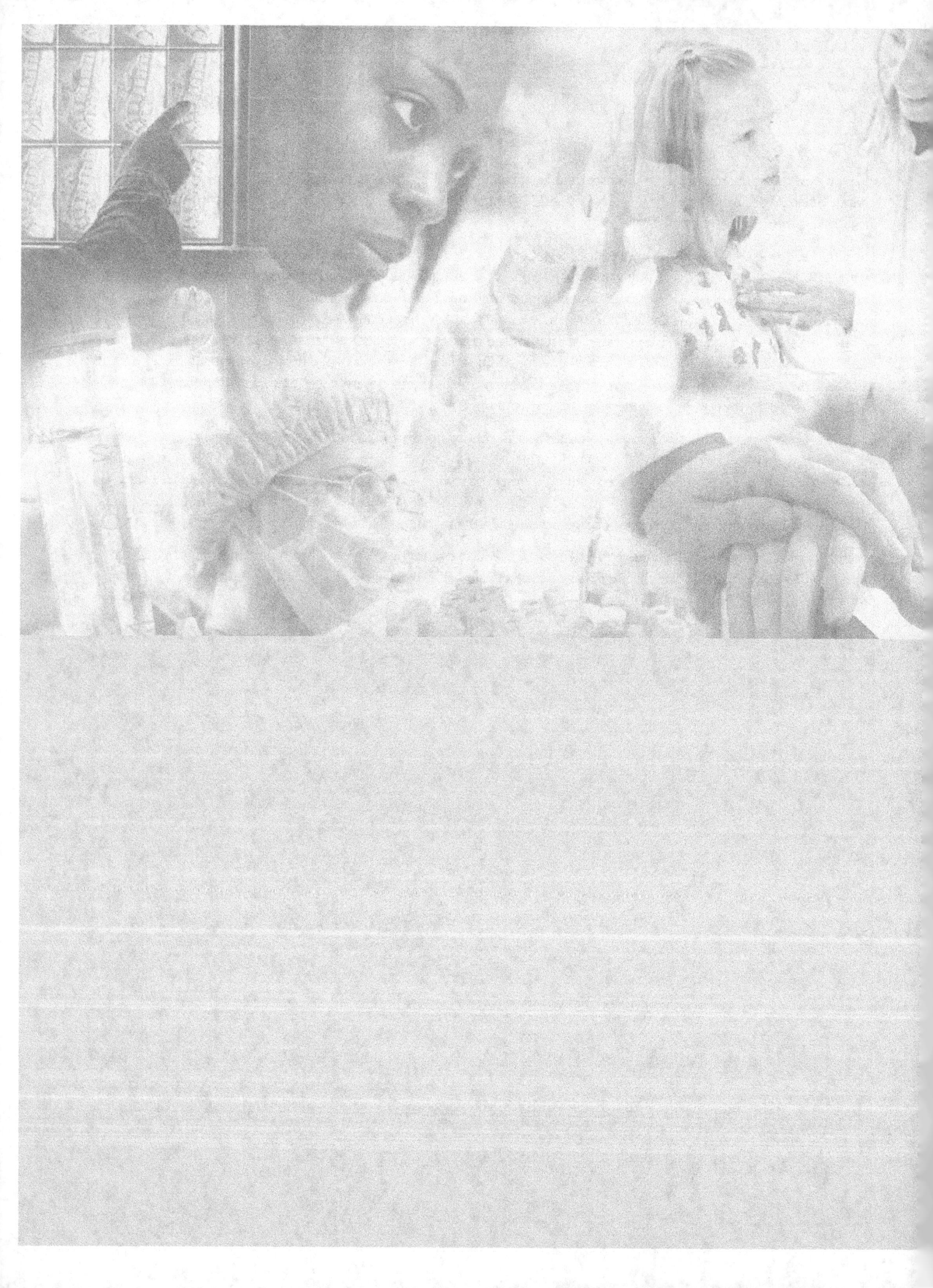

Introduction

Protecting the critical infrastructure and key resources (CIKR) of the United States is essential to the Nation's security, economic vitality, and way of life. Natural disasters, pandemics, terrorist attacks, and other manmade disasters—referred to collectively as "all hazards"—can significantly disrupt the functioning of government and business alike and produce cascading effects far beyond the physical location of the incident. The protection of the Nation's CIKR, therefore, is an essential part of the homeland security mission of making America safer, more secure, and more resilient in the face of all hazards. Protection includes actions to guard or shield CIKR assets, systems, networks, or their inter-connecting links from exposure, injury, destruction, incapacitation, or exploitation. This includes actions to deter, mitigate, or neutralize the threat, vulnerability, or consequences associated with all hazards. Protection consists of a wide range of activities, including hardening facilities, building resilience and redundancy, and implementing cybersecurity measures.

The National Infrastructure Protection Plan (NIPP) provides the framework for the cooperation that is needed to develop, implement, and maintain a coordinated national effort that brings together government at all levels, the private sector, and international organizations and allies. The NIPP provides a consistent, unifying structure for integrating CIKR protection efforts. It also provides the core processes and mechanisms to enable government and private sector partners to work together to implement CIKR protection initiatives. The cornerstone of the NIPP is its risk management framework, which establishes the processes for combining consequence, vulnerability, and threat information to produce a comprehensive, systematic, and rational assessment of national or sector risk. Figure I-1 depicts the NIPP risk management framework.

Figure I-1: NIPP Risk Management Framework

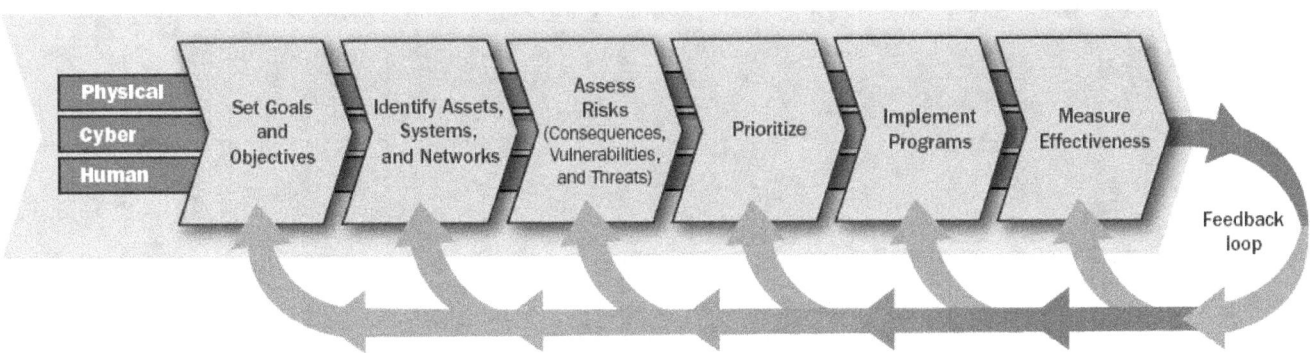

Continuous improvement to enhance protection of CIKR

Homeland Security Presidential Directive 7 (HSPD-7) and subsequent actions divide the national infrastructure into 18 CIKR sectors and assign protection responsibilities to selected Federal agencies, called Sector-Specific Agencies (SSAs). The U.S. Department of Health and Human Services (HHS) is the designated SSA for the Healthcare and Public Health (HPH) Sector. As the SSA, HHS is responsible for working with its sector partners to develop and maintain a Sector-Specific Plan (SSP) that details the application of the NIPP risk management framework to the unique characteristics and risk landscape of the HPH Sector.

1. Sector Profile and Goals

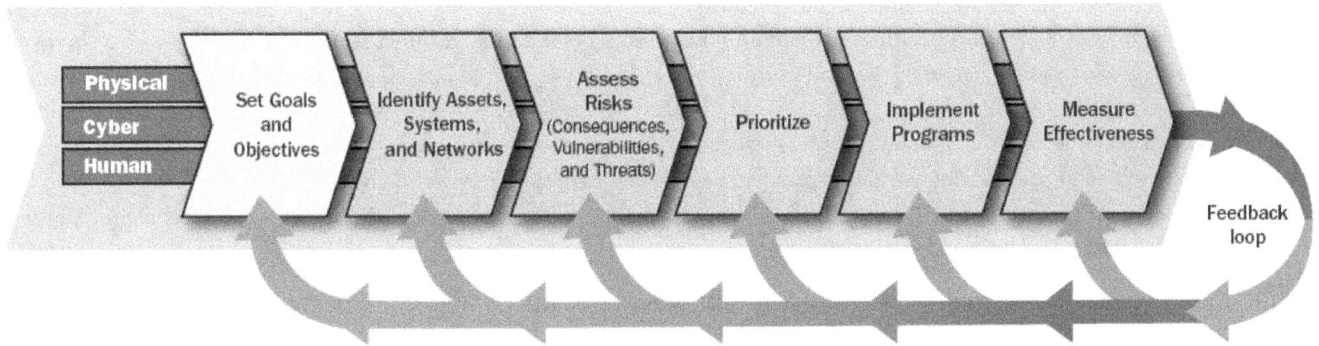

Continuous improvement to enhance protection of CIKR

This chapter provides a profile of the HPH Sector; a summary-level discussion about the sector's partners; the sector's vision, mission, goals, and objectives; and the value proposition that attracts the participation of sector organizations.

1.1 Sector Profile

The HPH Sector constitutes a significant portion of the U.S. economy. The U.S. Department of Health and Human Services estimates that 16.2 percent ($2.2 trillion) of our Nation's 2007 Gross Domestic Product (GDP) was spent on healthcare and forecasts this percentage to increase to 17.6 percent in 2009[1]. Privately owned and operated organizations comprise the vast majority of the sector and identify themselves with the delivery of healthcare goods and services. The public health component largely comprises government agencies at the Federal, State, local, tribal, and territorial levels. The public health component deals with health at the population level and has taken a lead role in large-scale disaster preparedness.

The HPH Sector provides a diverse array of goods and services that are distributed widely across the country. It includes not only acute care hospitals and ambulatory healthcare, but also the vast and complex public-private systems that finance that care. It includes population-based care provided by health agencies at the Federal, State, local, tribal, and territorial levels, as well as other public health and disease surveillance functions. It incorporates a large system of private sector enterprises that manufacture, distribute, and sell drugs, vaccines, and medical supplies and equipment, as well as a network of small businesses that

---

[1] Department of Health and Human Services, Centers for Medicare and Medicaid Services, National Health Expenditure Data: http://www.cms.hhs.gov/NationalHealthExpendData.

provide mortuary services. All these goods and services are provided in and by means of a complex environment of research, regulation, finance, and public policy.

The HPH Sector plays a crucial role in preparedness and response for all hazards. The sector is responsible for mitigating the physical and psychological health impacts associated with incidents. Sector partners plan collaboratively to ensure that the sector can provide needed services in the face of surging demand. Elements of the sector are present in virtually all U.S. communities at varying levels of capability. Although the sector does have several major, nationally organized entities, it is highly decentralized for the most part. Composed of both private and governmental entities, the boundaries between the two are often indistinguishable.

For the HPH Sector, critical infrastructure protection (CIP) is ultimately defined by the extent to which the sector has been able to mitigate interruptions in the delivery of healthcare and public health services. Among the challenges to implementing the CIP program in the sector are the breadth and diversity of the sector and the overlap between the sector's CIP role and its emergency response role.

There are approximately 13 million healthcare personnel[2] from many professions. Included are approximately five million first-responders with at least some emergency medical training, three million registered nurses, and more than 800,000 physicians. In alphabetical order, the overall figure includes, but is not limited to, the following personnel: behavioral health professionals; clinical laboratory technologists and technicians; emergency management specialists; emergency medical technicians and para-medics; firefighting occupations with medical capabilities; hazardous materials removal workers; nuclear medicine technolo-gists; nurses; occupational health and safety specialists; pharmacists; physicians; physician assistants; radiological technologists and technicians; respiratory therapists; and veterinarians.

Table 1-1 provides data that depict the size and breadth of the sector. It includes private sector and government data for comparison, where available.

---

[2] See Department of Health and Human Services, Health Resources and Services Administration. National Center for Health Workforce Analysis **http://bhpr.hrsa.gov/healthworkforce/reports**.

Table 1-1: Healthcare and Public Health Sector Statistics

Major Element	Private Sector	Public Sector			
		Federal	State	Local	Tribal
Healthcare personnel	> 13,000,000	> 450,000[a]			
Hospitals	3,905[b]	213[c]	1,105[d]		44[e]
Ambulatory healthcare services	~545,000 (unable to separate by ownership)[f]				
Nursing and residential care facilities	~75,000 (unable to separate by ownership)[g]				
Retail pharmacies	~42,000[h]				
Health departments		Parts of Federal departments and agencies, including HHS, Environmental Protection Agency, DoD, and VA	57	~3,000	36
Pharmaceutical manufacturers	~1,100[i]				
Medical device and supply companies	~ 2,500[j]				
Blood and organ banks	~1,200[k]				
Health insurers and other payers	>1,300[l]	1	50		

[a] See HHS, Health Resources and Services Administration, The Public Health Workforce Enumeration, **http://ask.hrsa.gov/detail_materials. cfm?ProdID=1057**.

[b] See American Hospital Association 2008 Survey Statistics.

[c] Ibid.

[d] Ibid.

[e] See Indian Health Services 2009 Fact Sheets.

[f] See U.S. Census Bureau, 2007 Economic Census, **http://www.census.gov/econ/census07**.

[g] Ibid.

[h] Ibid.

[i] Pharmaceutical manufacturers include pharmaceutical preparation manufacturers and medicinal and botanical manufacturers. See U.S. Census Bureau, 2007 Economic Census, **http://www.census.gov/econ/census07**.

[j] See U.S. Census Bureau, 2007 Economic Census, **http://www.census.gov/econ/census07**.

[k] Ibid.

[l] See America's Health Insurance Plans Association, **www.ahip.org**.

1.1.1 Significant Dependencies

The HPH Sector cannot sustain operations without the services provided by many of the other sectors. Table 1-2 describes the dependencies that the HPH Sector has on other sectors.

Table 1-2: Sector Dependencies

Sector	HPH Sector Dependency
Transportation	Movement of supplies, raw materials, pharmaceuticals, personnel, emergency response units, patients, and fatalities
Communications	Radio and telephone communications supporting a wide variety of business processes
Energy	Electric, natural gas, propane, and diesel fuel to power and run facility functions and vehicles
Water	Healthcare, pharmaceutical operations, and sanitation services
Emergency Services	Coordination with first-responders and emergency medical services; includes local law enforcement for security for various emergencies
Information Technology	Business and clinical information systems
Postal and Shipping	Movement of equipment and supplies
Chemical	Support to the pharmaceutical industry
Food and Agriculture	Food production and distribution for healthcare and public health personnel and patients

All other sectors are dependent on the HPH Sector to provide healthcare services to their workforce to sustain operations.

1.1.2 Significant Overlaps

Some functions in the HPH Sector overlap with functions of the Emergency Services, Food and Agriculture, Water, Chemical, and Commercial Facilities Sectors. Health agencies share responsibility with these sectors for protecting public health. The HPH and Emergency Services Sectors share responsibility for emergency preparedness and response. The HPH Sector works with the Food and Agriculture and Water Sectors to manage the safety of the nation's food and water supply. Pharmaceutical manufacturers in the HPH Sector also fall in the Chemical Sector and are governed by its regulations. Many facilities in the HPH Sector are also part of the Commercial Facilities Sector. Recognizing these overlaps, HHS continues to work closely with DHS to ensure a unified approach to CIKR protection issues across sectors.

1.1.3 Authorities Governing the Sector

Organizations in the sector are subject to a wide range of legislative and regulatory authorities. These authorities and constraints exist at the Federal, State, and local levels. The key authorities governing CIP in the sector include the following:

- **HSPD-7, section 18(b)**—Establishes the national framework for CIP and designates HHS as the SSA for healthcare, public health, and food (other than meat, poultry, and egg products).[3]

- **Pandemic and All-Hazards Preparedness Act**—Establishes in HHS an Assistant Secretary for Preparedness and Response (ASPR); authorizes or re-authorizes the key Federal programs for public health and medical preparedness; and calls for the establishment of a quadrennial National Health Security Strategy.

---

[3] Coordination of Sector-Specific Agency (SSA) responsibilities for the HPH Sector occurs in the HHS Office of the Assistant Secretary for Preparedness and Response. Coordination of SSA responsibilities for the food supply, excluding meat, poultry, and egg products, occurs in the HHS Food and Drug Administration. SSA responsibilities for meat, poultry, and egg products are coordinated by the U.S. Department of Agriculture.

- **Emergency Support Function 8 (ESF-8), Health and Medical Services Annex**—Provides the mechanism for coordinated Federal assistance to supplement State, local, tribal, and territorial resources in response to a public health and medical disaster, potential or actual incidents requiring a coordinated Federal response, and during a developing potential health and medical emergency. The Secretary of HHS, through the ASPR, coordinates national ESF-8 preparedness, response, and recovery actions.

- **HSPD-21**—Establishes a National Strategy for Public Health and Medical Preparedness to plan and enable provision for the public health and medical needs of the American people in a catastrophic health incident.

Appendix 2 lists these and other authorities governing the sector.

1.2 Sector Partners

Government and private sector entities share responsibility for protecting the HPH infrastructure. As the SSA, HHS is responsible for coordinating the participation of private sector, Federal, State, local, tribal, and territorial stakeholders in the CIP program. HHS accomplishes this task through its Sector Coordinating Council (SCC), Government Coordinating Council (GCC), relationships with the U.S. Department of Homeland Security (DHS) and other Federal departments and agencies, and participation in cross-sector groups and regional coalitions.

1.2.1 Coordinating Councils

The NIPP provides a framework for enhancing CIP through public-private partnership. The SCC, GCC, and joint work groups formed under the auspices of the Critical Infrastructure Partnership Advisory Council (CIPAC) are elements of this partnership model. Chapter 8 describes CIPAC and the implementation of the NIPP partnership model in detail.

Sector Coordinating Council

The Health SCC is a self-governing body representing the health industry that provides a forum for the private sector to discuss infrastructure protection issues and communicate with government. The SCC has organized itself in six subcouncils that represent many healthcare subsectors. These subcouncils and the types of organizations that belong in each are listed below:

- **Direct Health Care**—Healthcare systems, doctors' associations, nurses' associations, and medical facilities;

- **Health Information and Medical Technology**—Medical research institutions, information standards bodies, and electronic medical records system vendors;

- **Health Plans and Payers**—Health insurance companies and plans;

- **Mass Fatality Management**—Cemetery, cremation, and funeral home associations;

- **Medical Materials**—Medical equipment and supply manufacturers and distributors; and

- **Pharmaceuticals/Laboratories/Blood**—Pharmaceutical manufacturers, drug store chains, pharmacists' associations, laboratory associations, and blood banks.

The Federal Government uses the SCC as an entry point to the private sector to discuss and collaborate on CIP activities. Organizations represented on the SCC are listed in appendix 3.

Government Coordinating Council

The HPH GCC is the public sector component of the sector's public-private partnership framework. The objective of the GCC is to provide effective coordination of HPH CIP strategies and activities, policy, and communication across government and between the government and the private sector. The GCC includes representatives from across Federal, State, local, tribal, and territorial governments. HHS, as the SSA for the sector, chairs the GCC, and the DHS Office of Infrastructure Protection (IP) serves as co-chair.

HHS works through two major State and local healthcare and public health professional associations to establish appropriate links with State, local, and territorial public health entities. The National Association of County and City Health Officials (NACCHO) and the Association of State and Territorial Health Officials (ASTHO) have long-standing relationships with both HHS and their respective members. The SSA has been effective in forming relationships with both organizations, which are represented on the GCC. The SSA also works directly with several State Directors of Public Health and Preparedness (DPHPs) and benefits from their unique perspective and valuable contributions. The SSA will continue to reach out to States, localities, tribes, and Territories to increase their participation in the CIP program.

The organizations represented on the GCC are listed in appendix 4.

Joint Work Groups

The SCC and GCC work together closely and have formed many joint work groups in the CIPAC construct. This approach has proved very effective in accomplishing sector goals and objectives. Current work groups include the Information Sharing Work Group (ISWG), Joint Advisory Work Group (JAWG) for research and development (R&D) and modeling, simulation, and analysis (MS&A), Risk Assessment Work Group (RAWG), Cyber Security Work Group (CSWG), and Sector Annual Report (SAR) Writing Work Group. All work groups are designed to maximize participation from the private sector and State, local, tribal, and territorial partners. Chapter 8 provides further information on the creation of work groups in the sector.

1.2.2 Department of Homeland Security

As co-chairs of the GCC, HHS and DHS continually communicate and coordinate on HPH Sector CIP activities. HHS works with DHS to implement various presidential directives, executive orders, and statutes. The HPH CIP Program Manager holds monthly meetings that include DHS-assigned sector specialists, coordinating council secretariats, and other DHS support staff. These meetings help ensure that SSA and DHS resources are working together efficiently and effectively.

The HPH Sector works closely with the DHS Science and Technology (S&T) Directorate to exchange information on R&D priorities and needs for a wide range of research areas. The sector also coordinates with DHS to review threat information and provide insight on its vulnerabilities and the consequences that could result from all-hazards events.

HHS also works directly with various offices in DHS to fulfill its disaster preparedness and response missions to all-hazards events.

1.2.3 Other Federal Partners

The Department of Veterans Affairs (VA) and the Department of Defense (DoD) both operate vast healthcare and public health programs.

In VA, the Veterans Health Administration (VHA) operates the Nation's largest integrated health care system, overseeing the health care needs of millions of veterans. With a medical care appropriation of more than $47 billion, VHA employs more than 239,000 staff at more than 1,400 sites, including hospitals, clinics, and nursing homes.[4] In addition, VHA is the Nation's largest provider of graduate medical education and a major contributor to medical research.

---

[4] About VHA - **http://www1.va.gov/health/aboutVHA.asp**.

DoD operates the Military Health System (MHS), delivering healthcare to millions of DoD service members, retirees, and their families. MHS employs more than 135,000 staff and operates 63 hospitals and 413 medical clinics.[5] In addition to its healthcare services, MHS has full capability to respond to natural disasters and humanitarian crises around the globe.

HHS works closely with the VA and DoD to meet the sector's CIP goals. Through participation in the GCC and sector CIPAC work groups, the VA and DoD share best practices in CIP with other government entities and organizations in the private sector. VA and DoD also share population health data that support disease surveillance and subsequent workforce protection efforts. Both departments play a significant role in disaster planning and response activities.

The HPH SSA also works closely with DoD's Defense Critical Infrastructure Program Health Sector Working Group to maximize synergies among various components of each of their programs.

1.2.4 Cross-Sector Groups and Regional Coalitions

Members of the HPH Sector interact with other sectors through participation in cross-sector work groups, membership on the GCCs of other sectors, and monthly informal discussions with representatives from other sectors. HPH representatives participate in several DHS-led cross-sector groups, including the Cross-Sector Cyber Security Working Group (CSCSWG), the Cross-Sector R&D Work Group, and the Cross-Sector Education, Training, and Outreach Awareness Working Group. The HPH Sector also belongs to the GCCs for the Emergency Services, Food and Agriculture, and Water Sectors. HPH representatives meet monthly with representatives from the Food and Agriculture, Water, Energy, Defense Industrial Base, and Financial Services sectors to discuss a range of CIP topics. These interactions improve collaboration and coordination across sectors.

States have initiated several regional coalitions for collaboration on preparedness and response activities. As the lead agency for ESF-8, HHS participates in a number of these regional coalitions in support of its role in emergency preparedness and response. These coalitions include the All-Hazards Consortium[6] in the Mid-Atlantic and the Unified Planning Coalition[7] in the Southeast. HHS has staffed Regional Emergency Coordinators (RECs) in each of the Federal Emergency Management Agency (FEMA) regions to ensure strong collaboration between the Federal Government and the regions.

1.3 Sector Vision, Mission, Goals and Objectives

The vision for the HPH Sector is to achieve overall resilience against all hazards. Its mission is to sustain the essential functions of the Nation's healthcare and public health delivery system in times of crisis.

---

[5] Basic Facts of the Military Health System - http://www.tricare.mil/stakeholders/statistics.cfm.

[6] Details on the All Hazards Consortium can be found at http://www.ahcusa.org/index.htm.

[7] Details on the Unified Planning Coalition can be found at http://www.medicalreservecorps.gov/File/MRC_Resources/RegionIV/Conference/2007/RegionIV_UPC_Overview.pdf.

Figure 1-1: HPH Sector Vision and Mission

HPH Sector Vision Statement:

The HPH Sector will achieve overall resilience against all hazards. It will prevent or minimize damage to, or destruction of, the Nation's healthcare and public health infrastructure. It will strive to protect its workforce and preserve its ability to mount timely and effective responses, without disruption to services in non-impacted areas, and its ability to recover from both routine and emergency situations.

HPH Sector Mission Statement:

The mission of the HPH Sector is to sustain the essential functions of the Nation's healthcare and public health delivery system and to support effective emergency preparedness and response to nationally significant hazards by implementing strategies, evaluating risks, coordinating plans and policy advice, and providing guidance to prepare, protect, prevent, and, when necessary, respond to attacks on the Nation's infrastructure and ensure the necessary resilience in infrastructure to recover and reconstitute healthcare and public health.

To support its vision and mission, the sector has established goals and objectives in the areas of service continuity, workforce protection, physical asset protection, and cybersecurity. Table 1-3 describes these goals.

Table 1-3: HPH Sector Goals

Sector Goals	
Service Continuity	Maintain the ability to provide essential health services during and after disasters or disruptions in the availability of supplies or supporting services (e.g., water, power).
Workforce Protection	Protect the sector's workforce from the harmful consequences of all hazards that may compromise their health and safety and limit their ability to carry out their responsibilities.
Physical Asset Protection	Mitigate the risks posed by all hazards to the sector's physical assets.
Cybersecurity	Mitigate risks to the sector's cyber assets that may result in disruption to or denial of health services.

The HPH Sector has identified a series of objectives that support its service continuity, workforce protection, physical asset protection, and cybersecurity goals. These objectives serve to direct efforts in the sector to improve CIKR protection. Table 1-4 describes the objectives.

Table 1-4: HPH Sector Objectives

Service Continuity	
Health Care Continuity	Enhance the ability of healthcare facilities to provide care during all-hazards incidents.
Supply Chain Continuity	Mitigate the threat of disruptions in the supply of drugs, biological products, medical devices, and other critical supplies.
Supporting Services Continuity	Mitigate risks to the sector of disruptions in supporting services, including water, power, transportation, telecommunications, and waste management.
Workforce Family Member Protection	Plan for the protection of the sector's workforce family members to increase the availability of the workforce for emergency response.
CIKR Essential Personnel Protection	Assist other CIKR sectors in the protection of their essential personnel through public health measures.
Workforce Protection	
Mass Prophylaxis	Enhance protection of the sector's workforce through the availability and rapid delivery of countermeasures and protective equipment.
Health Surveillance	Improve and maintain health surveillance systems to enable the rapid and accurate detection of all-hazards events and monitoring of the associated health consequences.
Physical Asset Protection	
Biosafety Level (BSL) 3 and 4 Facility Protection	Mitigate risks posed to Biosafety Level 3 and 4 facilities that use select agents so that harmful biological agents and toxins are secured and laboratory services are available for response.
Countermeasure Facility Security	Enhance the security of facilities involved in the development and stockpiling of medical countermeasures.
Healthcare and Public Health Facility Protection	Improve the sector's ability to protect against direct threats to healthcare and public health facilities posed by all hazards.
Research Facility Protection	Mitigate risks posed by all hazards to the sector's critical research facilities.
Cybersecurity	
Cyber Network, System, and Data Protection	Protect against cyber attacks that disrupt or compromise critical information technology networks, systems, and data supporting the sector.

The SSA, SCC, and GCC will continue to evaluate the sector's mission, vision, goals, and objectives annually to ensure that they are aligned with the NIPP and remain current as the sector's CIP program continues to mature.

1.4 Value Proposition

The engagement of sector owners and operators in the CIP program is crucial to achieving a more prepared and resilient sector. HHS strives to ensure that owners and operators who participate in the program find value that justifies their investment of time and resources.

Organizations that participate in the program gain access to security resources. HHS makes a wide range of products and services available to the sector, including online tools, safety guides, secure communication channels, and incident alerts and conference calls. Using these products and services keeps organizations up-to-date on the latest security issues, promoting an informed and secure sector.

Participation in the CIP program offers organizations the ability to maintain awareness of threats and make more informed decisions. As a result, they can more effectively reduce their vulnerability, mitigate business risk, and improve enterprise resilience. HHS has taken an aggressive approach to broaden the sharing of classified information with State, local, tribal, territorial, and private sector partners. The SSA, with the assistance of DHS, obtains security clearances for State, local, tribal, territorial, and private sector personnel participating in various joint working groups and conducts several briefings a year for partners with the appropriate security clearances.

Owners and operators also have the opportunity to collaborate with and learn from each other, promulgating best practices across the sector. They may use their participation to gain support and engagement in their own voluntary CIP activities. The CIP program provides participating organizations with a platform to voice their opinions and needs, enhancing government policies, plans, and actions on infrastructure protection.

Implementation Steps: Developing Sector Profile and Goals

The profile and goals of the HPH Sector will vary, depending on a particular organization's unique situation. In embarking on a critical infrastructure protection program in a State, local, tribal, territorial, or private sector organization, it is helpful to define the organization's perspective on *what* is to be protected, *who* are the key stakeholders, and *how* they will work together to establish and implement goals and objectives. These are the steps to develop a sector profile and goals:

- Research and describe the healthcare and public health sector in your jurisdiction.

- Identify critical infrastructure protection partners.

- Develop a plan for critical infrastructure protection.

For additional implementation considerations related to these steps, please see appendix 5.

---

2. Identify Assets, Systems, and Networks

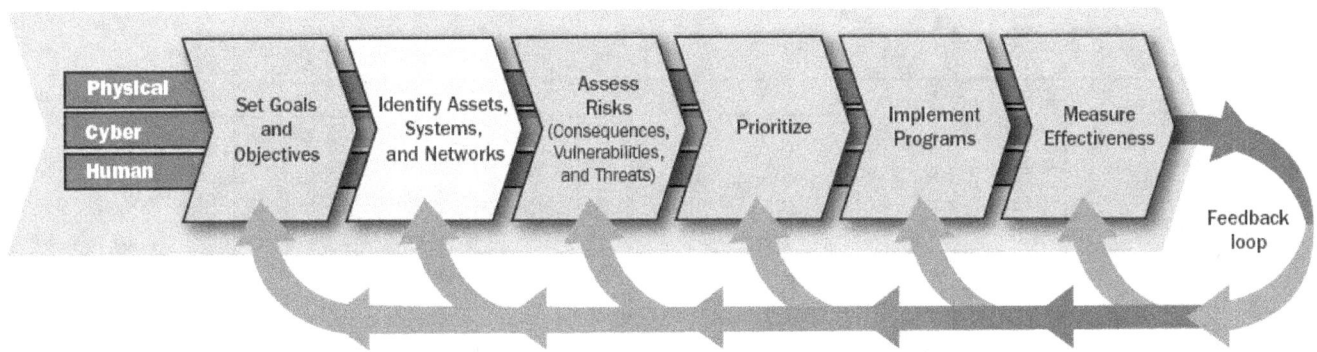

Continuous improvement to enhance protection of CIKR

This chapter discusses the HPH Sector's process for identifying critical assets, systems, and networks. It describes the sector's framework for critical infrastructure identification and the sector's approach to collecting and verifying information about critical infrastructure.

2.1 Defining Information Parameters

In the fall of 2007, the SSA initiated a functional analysis of the HPH Sector. Sector subject matter experts identified sector domains[8] and capabilities,[9] forming a hierarchical structure within which to identify, define, and organize sector functions[10] in a functional model. Following this work, the SSA convened panels of experts to define functions for capabilities in the population health management and emergency management domains. During the fall of 2009, work resumed on the functional model, and the SSA convened subject matter experts to define the functions that support the capabilities of the medical supply chain domain.

The functional model provides a framework for identifying assets, systems, and networks. With the model, the sector has the ability to evaluate functions and determine the underlying infrastructure necessary to support these functions. As an example, the performance of the public health surveillance function depends on cyber systems, like the Centers for Disease Control and

---

[8] The sector defines a domain as a set of services in a sector that share a common mission or purpose. A domain comprises multiple capabilities.

[9] The sector defines a capability as the ability to perform designated activities that fulfill a given set of requirements in a sector's domain. A capability comprises multiple functions.

[10] The sector defines a function as a set of activities or operations that are carried out to provide sector goods or services.

Prevention's (CDC) BioSense, which gather and analyze clinical data to identify potential disease outbreaks. The functional model enables the sector to view its infrastructure from a business continuity perspective. The sector will continue to use this approach as a framework for identifying assets, systems, and networks.

2.2 Collecting Infrastructure Information

In accordance with the 9/11 Commission Act, DHS is the lead coordinator in the national effort to identify and prioritize the Nation's CIKR. DHS executes this responsibility through the National Critical Infrastructure Prioritization Program (NCIPP).[11] Through this program, the sectors and States identify domestic infrastructure which, if disrupted, could critically impact the Nation's public health and safety, economy, or national security. Preparation of the list of these assets includes an evaluation process that prioritizes assets at four levels. The resulting lists of prioritized assets inform grant programs and are used during incidents for prioritizing Federal, State, and local response and recovery efforts. Figure 2-2 depicts the prioritization process.

Figure 2-2: The DHS Data Call Process

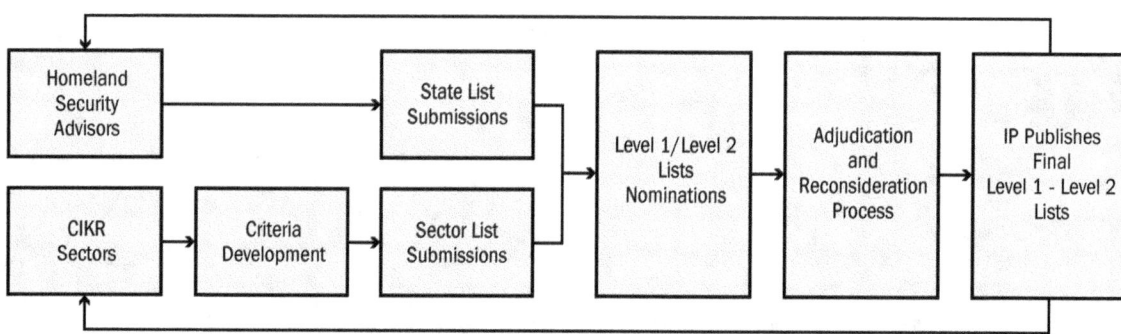

The HPH Sector fully participates in NCIPP through its RAWG. Comprising experts from across the sector, this work group is responsible for developing and refining the sector's critical infrastructure identification criteria. The RAWG analyzes critical functions in the sector which, if disrupted, would lead to overall mission degradation and cascading consequences. The group then identifies asset types that support these critical functions and their associated attributes. This information forms the basis for developing the criteria. Using this approach, the HPH Sector has defined criteria for eight asset types that provide critical steady-state and emergency response capabilities. The RAWG will continue to perform this function, annually reviewing and refining the sector's criteria.

Collecting the necessary information on critical infrastructure in the sector requires a collaborative effort. DHS works with State Homeland Security Advisors (HSAs), providing them with the criteria and assisting them in the creation and submission of the list of qualifying assets. The SSA assists the process by informing the DPHPs in State health agencies about NCIPP and providing them with the criteria so that they can help their State HSAs identify health-related infrastructure. In the coming years, the RAWG plans to increase its involvement in NCIPP, with a focus on collecting asset information for the sector list.

Current and accurate information on critical infrastructure is essential to the success of the CIP program. The sector uses information from data calls to identify hazards and vulnerabilities, analyze sector functions and capabilities, and prioritize assets and systems. By providing a high level of protection for infrastructure information, the SSA can encourage more robust information sharing among sector partners.

---

[11] This program is commonly referred to as Level 1, Level 2 Asset Identification.

The Homeland Security Act created a category of information which, when submitted to the Federal Government by private sector entities, can be protected from public disclosure under the Freedom of Information Act (FOIA), State and local sunshine laws, and civil litigation proceedings. This information is called Protected Critical Infrastructure Information (PCII).[12] Final rules for handling such information are contained in Procedures for Handling Critical Infrastructure Information.[13] These procedures govern the receipt, validation, handling, storage, marking, and use of critical infrastructure information voluntarily submitted to the Federal Government. The procedures are applicable to all Federal, State, local, tribal, and territorial government agencies, and contractors that have access to, handle, use, or store critical infrastructure information that is protected under the Critical Infrastructure Information (CII) Act of 2002. The HPH Sector works closely with DHS to ensure adherence to all regulations regarding PCII.

2.3 Verifying and Updating Infrastructure Information

The sector reviews asset information for accuracy and completeness as part of its participation in NCIPP. As depicted in figure 2-2, all data call submissions are subject to an adjudication and reconsideration process. The SSA uses the criteria to review State submissions for applicability, accuracy, and completeness, and works with DHS and the States to determine the final priority lists of HPH assets. The HPH Sector will continue to participate in NCIPP to maintain its list of critical assets.

2.4 The Path Forward

The HPH Sector continues to mature in its ability to effectively identify its critical assets, systems, and networks. The sector will continue to conduct its functional analysis to support identification of the underlying infrastructure necessary to perform critical functions. The sector will increase RAWG involvement in NCIPP, fully engaging the work group in the information collection and verification processes. The sector will also develop a more formal list of assets that do not qualify for Level 1/Level 2 designation, but which are still deemed important or critical to the sector.

Implementation Steps: Identifying Assets, Systems, and Networks

The HPH Sector comprises many diverse elements. A thorough process is required to identify the assets, systems, and networks that comprise the sector. These are the steps to identify sector elements:

- Identify healthcare and public health critical infrastructure for your entity or jurisdiction.

- Take a broad approach in identifying critical assets and systems.

- Become involved in national and jurisdictional data calls for critical infrastructure and key resources.

For additional implementation considerations related to these steps, please see appendix 5.

---

[12] See Homeland Security Act of 2002, 6 United States Code (U.S.C.) 133, Section 214.

[13] See Federal Register, September 1, 2006 (Vol. 71, No. 170), DHS, Office of the Secretary, Procedures for Handling Critical Infrastructure Information, which establishes uniform procedures for implementing the Critical Infrastructure Information Act of 2002.

3. Assess Risks

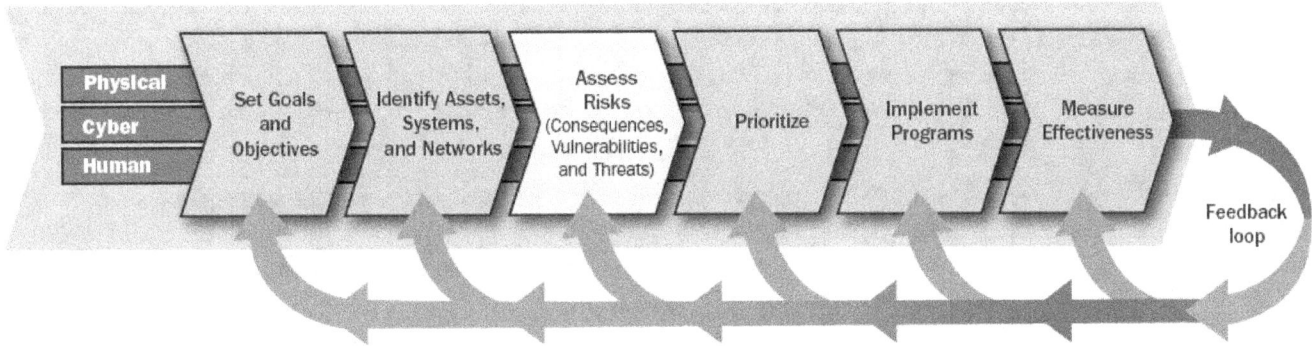

Continuous improvement to enhance protection of CIKR

This chapter provides information on the HPH Sector's approach for assessing risk. It includes information about some risk analysis tools and describes vulnerability and consequence assessment in the sector.

3.1 Use of Risk Assessment in the Sector

Most risk assessment performed in the HPH Sector is conducted to achieve compliance with safety, physical security, and information security regulations. Following are some examples:

- Hospitals must conduct risk assessments to meet State regulations and achieve certification required for reimbursement by the Federal Medicare program.

- Pharmaceutical manufacturers conduct risk assessments to meet regulations that ensure the efficacy of their products.

- Sector health plans, healthcare providers, and healthcare clearinghouses assess risks to systems that maintain health data to ensure compliance with security and privacy rules in the Health Insurance Portability and Accountability Act (HIPAA) of 1996.

- Federal partners conduct risk assessments as a component of the certification and accreditation process to comply with the Federal Information Security Management Act (FISMA) of 2002.

Beyond the need to meet regulatory requirements, HPH Sector organizations have a vested interest in conducting risk assessment to identify risks that could lead to negative financial consequences and damage to their reputations. The SSA will assist sector partners with this process by identifying and sharing risk assessment tools.

3.2 Assessing Vulnerabilities and Consequences

Organizations in the HPH Sector use various tools and methods to assess vulnerabilities and consequences. This section focuses on the vulnerability and consequence assessment activities led by the SSA, SCC, and GCC partnership.

3.2.1 Strategic Homeland Infrastructure Risk Analysis

The Strategic Homeland Infrastructure Risk Analysis (SHIRA), led by the Homeland Infrastructure Threat and Risk Analysis Center (HITRAC), establishes a common framework that sectors can use to assess the economic, loss of life, and psychological consequences resulting from terrorist incidents. The model has matured over time, incorporating natural hazards and domestic threats, to help sectors characterize vulnerabilities to and consequences that result from all hazards.

On behalf of the HPH Sector, the RAWG uses the SHIRA methodology to develop scenarios of real-world events that could impact critical sector services, including the delivery of care and the medical supply chain. To date, the RAWG has developed scenarios that depict vulnerabilities and consequences related to biological, cyber, vehicle-born explosive device, and insider threats. The analysis favors those events that are high consequence and have a possibility of occurring. Representative targets include laboratories handling biological select agents and toxins, manufacturing facilities, medical supply storage facilities, and cyber infrastructure. The resulting data enable sector subject matter experts to examine complex cascading consequences for economic, loss of life, and psychological impacts.

The sector uses the data generated by the SHIRA process to inform other CIP-related efforts, including the development of capability gap statements for research and development investments and the creation of critical infrastructure criteria for the NCIPP. The sector will continue to leverage SHIRA to guide protection and consequence reduction decisions and to improve overall mission effectiveness.

3.2.2 Network Analysis

The HPH CIP program is conducting a network analysis of the sector to gain a more detailed understanding of sector risk. This approach makes use of the sector's functional model (described in chapter 2) to examine sector interdependencies, external dependencies, and critical nodes. The process exposes underlying vulnerabilities and potential points of failure, and enables the sector to analyze cascading consequences that result from the failure of a function and develop risk management strategies. Leveraging this effort, the sector can integrate modeling and simulation of varying scenarios at the national, regional, or local level to develop mitigation strategies; enhance protective programs; direct resource allocation; and identify gaps in services associated with emergency response, recovery, health surveillance, and the delivery of care.

3.2.3 Healthcare Facility Risk and Design Analysis Tool

The HPH Sector is developing a healthcare facility security and design analysis tool for use by building owners and designers. The tool analyzes the security risks of a facility based on geographic location, natural hazards, and service types to facilitate optimal design options for security and medical surge. An organization using the tool answers a series of questions about facility attributes, threat characteristics, historical risk assessments, and safety and security features. The tool aggregates and synthesizes the responses to provide a total facility risk score. As the tool matures, each question will be linked to a series of mitigation strategies that are recommended for consideration in the design or remodeling of the facility. The results of the analysis are intended for use by owners and operators, as well as architects to inform design decisions at the onset of a project. The benefits of integrating security during the design phase of building include reduced costs related to purchasing and integration, improved patient and workforce safety during surge, and enhanced operational sustainability during an all-hazards incident.

3.2.4 Cybersecurity Risk Assessment

The HPH Sector formed the CSWG to develop a strategy for improving cybersecurity in the sector. The effort has received significant support from the vendor community, cross-sector cyber experts, and owners and operators. The CSWG has created a framework to categorize cyber risks based on the loss of system availability, data integrity, confidentiality, or privacy. In these risk categories, the CSWG has analyzed threats, vulnerabilities, consequences, cascading consequences, and mitigation strategies. Table 3-1 provides more detail.

Table 3-1: Common Cyber Threats, Vulnerabilities, Consequences, and Mitigation Strategies

Category	Common Elements
Threats	Insider threat, hacking, and terrorism Botnets, malware, phishing, and distributed denial of service Natural disaster
Vulnerabilities	Inadequate patch management, configuration management, and password management Lack of antivirus protection and intrusion prevention and protection Software vulnerabilities and SQL injection Open USB ports and DVD, CD, and R/W drives
Consequences	Loss of personally identifying information and identity theft Patient errors Inability to use patient data or deliver HPH services
Cascading Consequences	Forensic and system recovery service fees Blackmail and fraud (medical and financial) Loss of brand reputation Civil suits Financial theft and insolvency Loss of services Loss of life
Mitigation Strategies	Redundant and failover systems and warm backup sites Background investigations Identity management Multifactor authentication Intrusion prevention and detection Least privilege Data encryption Anti-virus software Auditing Hardware lockdown

3.3 Path Forward

The HPH Sector will continue to build its risk assessment capability through the use of risk assessment tools and network analysis. The RAWG, with support from the SSA, will evaluate available risk assessment tools and educate members of the sector on their use. The SSA will also continue to extend the network analysis and leverage it to inform its risk mitigation activities.

Implementation Steps: Assessing Risk

The HPH Sector faces many different risks, some of which are unique to a particular jurisdiction or industry. A thorough risk analysis will address risks that are expected, as well as those that may occur infrequently. These are the steps to assess risks:

- Conduct a hazard vulnerability assessment.

- Match risks against protection goals and objectives.

For additional implementation considerations related to these steps, please see appendix 5.

---

4. Prioritize Infrastructure

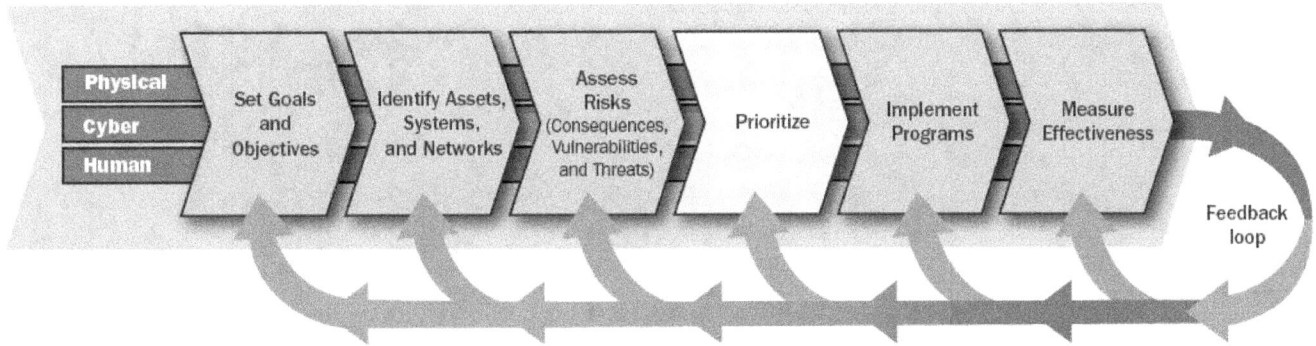

Continuous improvement to enhance protection of CIKR

Chapter 4 discusses the sector's current process and path forward for prioritizing its critical assets, systems, and networks.

4.1 Current Prioritization Process

The HPH Sector's current prioritization process occurs through its participation in the NCIPP. In partnership with the SSA, DHS conducts a consequence-based risk assessment to determine which critical assets are of national significance and which should be prioritized ahead of other sector assets. Chapter 2 provides a more thorough description of this process.

4.2 The Path Forward

Using the criteria it developed for NCIPP, the sector plans to expand its current prioritization process to include the formal identification of a third level of assets. The RAWG will lead this effort on behalf of the sector. Where prioritization at an asset, system, or network level is not possible, the sector will prioritize subsectors for specific threats. For example, the sector may prioritize the protection of health insurers from cyber attacks, hospitals from active shooters, and manufacturing facilities and transportation nodes from supply chain interruption. This approach will provide a sharper focus for the sector's CIP efforts.

Implementation Steps: Prioritizing Infrastructure

In the broad range of HPH Sector assets, systems, and networks that have been identified, certain infrastructure components would lead to the most severe consequences if compromised. After these components have been identified, an organization will be better equipped to prioritize resources and activities to protect the sector. This is the step for prioritizing infrastructure:

- Prioritize hazards and critical infrastructure based on probability and consequence.

For additional implementation considerations related to this step, please see appendix 5.

5. Develop and Implement Protective Programs and Resilience Strategies

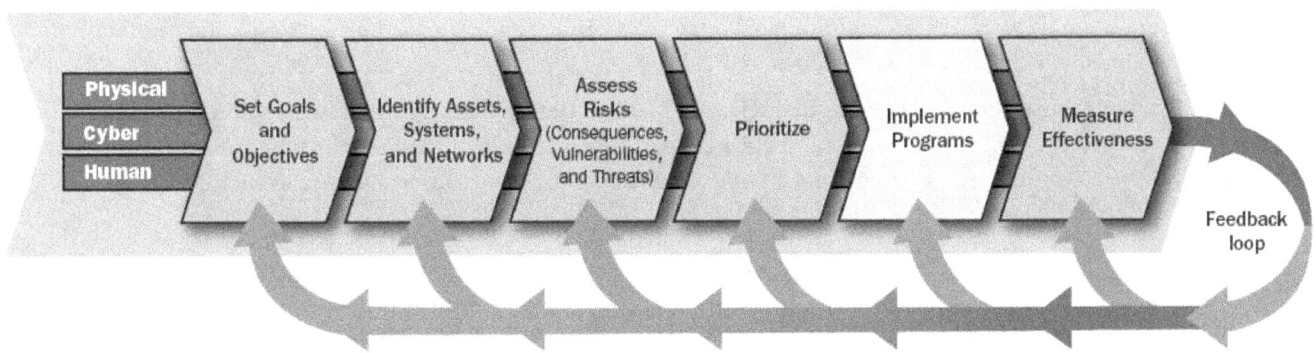

| Physical | Cyber | Human |

Set Goals and Objectives → Identify Assets, Systems, and Networks → Assess Risks (Consequences, Vulnerabilities, and Threats) → Prioritize → Implement Programs → Measure Effectiveness

Feedback loop

Continuous improvement to enhance protection of CIKR

This chapter describes some of the major protective programs and resilience strategies in the sector and the current processes for identifying CIP needs and implementing CIP programs.

5.1 Overview of Sector Protective Programs and Resilience Strategies

Government and private sector organizations develop and implement protective programs and resilience strategies to address a wide range of challenges that relate to the sector's goals. As the SSA, HHS facilitates communication between government and private sector organizations through the partnership model to increase collaboration and the effectiveness of the sector's protective programs and resilience strategies.

The following subsections describe several ongoing HPH Sector CIP programs and initiatives. These programs and initiatives are organized by the sector goals of service continuity, workforce protection, physical asset protection, and cybersecurity, and they correspond to the risk mitigation activities (RMAs) described in the 2009 HPH SAR.

Goal 1: Service Continuity

- **HHS Hospital Preparedness Program**—A Federal cooperative agreement program operated by HHS and administered through State, local, tribal, and territorial health agencies. This program enhances the ability of hospitals and healthcare systems to prepare for and respond to bioterrorism and other public health emergencies. Program priority areas include interoperable communication systems, bed tracking, personnel management, fatality management planning, and hospital evacuation planning.

- **The Joint Commission Healthcare Facility Accreditation Programs**—Offer hospital, ambulatory care, behavioral healthcare, home care, long-term care, and office-based surgery accreditation programs. These programs include standards that require healthcare facilities to plan for all hazards.

- **RxResponse**—A nonprofit, private sector initiative to support the medical supply chain during emergencies. RxResponse partners work together with Federal, State, and local officials, as well as with volunteer organizations to help support the continued delivery of medicines to people who need them in an emergency.

- **CDC Public Health Emergency Preparedness Cooperative Agreement, Preparedness, and Response Activities**—A Federal cooperative agreement program operated by HHS and administered through State, local, tribal, and territorial health agencies that provides funding to enable public health departments to have the capacity and capability to effectively respond to the public health consequences of all hazards.

- **Project Public Health Ready**—A competency-based training and recognition program that assesses preparedness and assists local health departments or groups of local health departments working collaboratively as a region to respond to emergencies. The program is funded by CDC and administered by the NACCHO. It builds preparedness capacity and capability through a continuous quality improvement model.

- **Food and Drug Administration (FDA) Drug, Biologic, and Medical Device Shortage Programs**—Address potential or actual shortages that have a significant impact on public health. Through communication, facilitation, and negotiation, these programs work with medical manufacturers and other government agencies to plan for and manage shortages of medically necessary products.

Goal 2: Workforce Protection

- **CDC Public Health Emergency Preparedness Cooperative Agreement, Disease Detection, and Investigation Activities**— Improves the ability of public health departments to detect and investigate diseases and increase their capacity for laboratory testing for bioterrorism agents. Through these funds, public health departments have increased the number of epidemiologists working in emergency response, the number of public health professionals using health surveillance systems, and the number of laboratories capable of testing for biological and chemical agents.

- **CDC Cities Readiness Initiative**—Provides funding and technical assistance to prepare major U.S. Metropolitan Statistical Areas (MSAs) to effectively respond to a large-scale bioterrorist attack by dispensing countermeasures to the affected population within 48 hours.

Goal 3: Physical Asset Protection

- **CDC Select Agent Program**—Regulates the possession, use, and transfer of biological agents and toxins that could pose a severe threat to public health and safety (known as select agents). This program promotes laboratory safety and security by developing, implementing, and enforcing the select agent regulations; providing guidance to the regulated community; and inspecting facilities working with select agents.

- **HHS Biomedical Advanced Research and Development Authority (BARDA) Program Protection Office (PPO)**— Establishes security standards, provides guidance, and ensures compliance throughout the complete life-cycle acquisition process of critical vaccines, diagnostics, and drugs acquired under PBS and the PIEID Program. PPO administers and ensures compliance with comprehensive security practices relating to physical security, operations security, personnel security, information security, and transportation security, and conducts security awareness programs at all contractor facilities supporting PBS and PIEID.

- **Hospital Protection Activities**—Federally funded programs designed to improve the ability of hospitals to protect against direct attacks and natural disasters. These programs include the Buffer Zone Protection Program and Protective Security Advisor Enhanced Critical Infrastructure Protection visits.

Goal 4: Cybersecurity

The HPH Sector participates in overarching Federal cybersecurity programs, including the CSCSWG. The sector also leads a number of cybersecurity initiatives unique to the HPH Sector. These initiatives are focused on developing standards for the secure exchange of health information across organizational boundaries.

- **HHS Nationwide Privacy and Security Framework**—Establishes a baseline of national privacy and security standards that apply to Individually Identifiable Health Information (IIHI) held by Federal, State, local, public, and private healthcare providers, plans, and clearinghouses.

- **The Health Information Technology Standards Panel (HITSP)**—Serves as a cooperative partnership between the public and private sectors to achieve a commonly accepted and useful set of standards to enable and support widespread interoperability, security, and privacy among healthcare software applications.

- **National Institute of Standards and Technology (NIST) Health Information Exchange (HIE) Standards**—Identify and establish standardized security controls for the exchange of protected health information, as defined under HIPAA, and develop a methodology to support the security architecture design of HIEs and Health Information Networks (HIN).

5.2 Determining the Need for Protective Programs and Resilience Strategies

Legislative and regulatory mandates drive many of the government programs and resilience strategies in the HPH Sector. Congress identifies CIP needs and creates Federal programs and strategies to address these needs. State, local, tribal, and territorial governments participate in Federal CIP programs, as do private sector organizations to the extent that these programs are required or meet their CIP needs.

State, local, territorial, and tribal governments also assess unique CIP needs in their jurisdictions and develop corresponding programs to address these needs. Private sector organizations may choose or be required to participate in these programs.

Many private sector organizations in the HPH Sector assess risks to their infrastructure as part of their business continuity programs. The organizations identify CIP needs based on these risk assessments and implement protective programs to address these needs.

At the SSA, the CIP Program Manager works with SCC leadership to set priorities for the program based on needs expressed by members of the SCC and GCC. These priorities often lead to the creation and implementation of initiatives to address the needs.

5.3 Protective Program/Resilience Strategy Implementation

Government and private sector organizations from across the HPH Sector implement protective programs and resilience strategies with varying degrees of coordination. The Federal Government implements large programs with participation from all levels of government and the private sector. Agencies responsible for these programs work in a collaborative fashion with other government and private sector entities to ensure that these programs benefit the sector. States, localities, tribes, and Territories implement protective programs in their jurisdictions in coordination with the Federal Government and private sector. Private sector organizations implement protective programs and resilience strategies that suit the unique aspects of their organizations. The SSA supports CIP programs at all levels in multiple ways, primarily by facilitating the sharing of information.

5.4 Monitoring Program Implementation

In the HPH Sector, government agencies and private sector organizations monitor their programs to varying degrees. Chapter 6 contains a more detailed description of these monitoring activities.

5.5 Path Forward

The HPH Sector will continue to foster an environment where public and private sector organizations can communicate about their programs and collaborate when possible to achieve maximum effectiveness. The sector will continue to inform senior officials involved in policy development so that their decisions take the most critical protection needs of the sector into consideration.

Implementation Steps: Developing and Implementing Protective Programs and Resilience Strategies

After critical infrastructure and key resources have been identified and prioritized, protection initiatives and resilience strategies may be developed and targeted to protect the sector as a whole. These are the steps to develop and implement protective programs and resilience strategies:

- Identify initiatives that are already underway.

- Identify protection gaps.

- Develop risk mitigation activities.

For additional implementation considerations related to these steps, please see appendix 5.

---

6. Measure Effectiveness

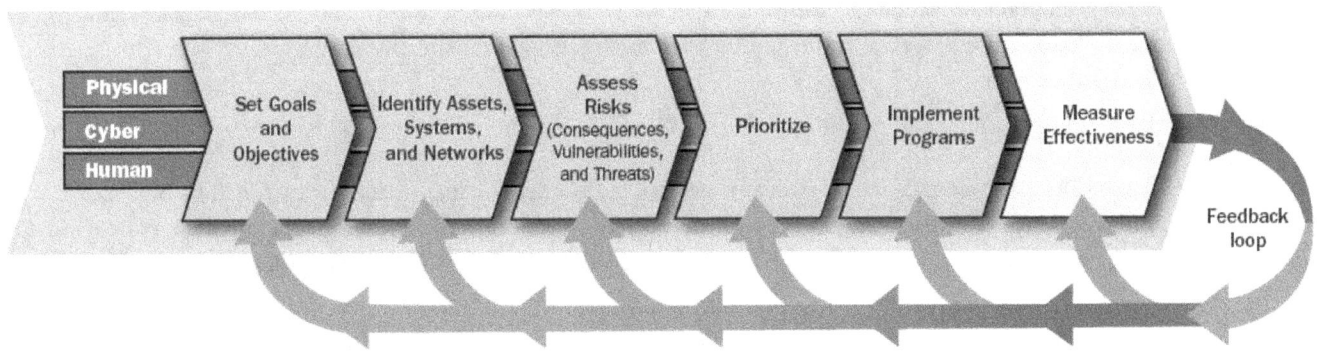

Continuous improvement to enhance protection of CIKR

This chapter provides information about the sector's key RMAs, processes for measuring effectiveness, and approach for using measurement to foster continuous improvement.

6.1 Risk Mitigation Activities

The HPH Sector identifies key RMAs based on their alignment with sector goals and their level of impact. Most of the sector's key RMAs are focused on service continuity. The sector has made significant investments in programs that improve its ability to continue delivering healthcare during and immediately following all-hazards events. The sector also has key RMAs that protect its workforce by improving health surveillance and mass prophylaxis capabilities. The sector has increased emphasis on RMAs that protect critical physical assets, with a focus on biosafety labs, hospitals, and sites where medical countermeasures are stockpiled. While the sector does not have key RMAs focused on cybersecurity yet, a number of programs and strategies in this area are underway and may become key RMAs in the future.

Detailed information about the sector's key RMAs is provided in the HPH SAR.

6.2 Process for Measuring Effectiveness

The HPH Sector relies on performance measurement done at the program level to indicate progress toward achieving its CIP goals and objectives. Most federally funded programs require grant awardees to report their progress annually. The agencies that manage these programs provide the CIP Program Office with this performance data for use in determining and reporting on progress. The SSA includes performance measurement information on the progress of key RMAs in its SAR.

The sector measures engagement in its CIP program. Metrics based on participation in CIP meetings, use of the sector's information-sharing portal, and participation in work groups provide meaningful information about the progress of the sector's CIP program. The sector will continue to monitor program engagement, with a focus on measuring information-sharing activities.

6.3 Using Metrics for Continuous Improvement

Increasingly, Federal agencies that fund and administer large CIP-related programs are basing future funding decisions on the performance of grant awardees. In some cases, a failure to meet program objectives is penalized by withholding funds during the current year. As program objectives are met, the Federal Government frequently raises the bar by setting higher standards and new objectives. This approach uses metrics to foster continuous improvement.

At the macro level, Congress, the Office of Management and Budget, and other Federal oversight organizations review the effectiveness of large CIP-related programs through Government Accountability Office studies, the use of the Program Assessment Rating Tool, and other program evaluation mechanisms. Based on the results of these assessments, the Federal Government may increase funding for effective programs and reduce or eliminate funding for ineffective programs.

6.4 Path Forward

Moving forward, the CIP Program Office will continue to leverage performance management data provided by organizations that fund large CIP programs to gauge the sector's progress in protecting its critical infrastructure. The program office will also work with these organizations to add measures to their performance management systems that are CIP-focused.

Implementation Steps: Measuring Effectiveness

HPH Sector organizations are often experienced with using data to inform clinical decisions or the implementation of public health programs. By measuring effectiveness of protection initiatives and resilience strategies, an organization can ensure that resources are being maximized to protect the sector as a whole. These are the steps to measure effectiveness:

- Identify measures of critical infrastructure protection.

- Identify data sources for measurement.

For additional implementation considerations related to these steps, please see appendix 5.

---

7. CIKR Protection Research & Development

This chapter describes the HPH Sector's approach to managing its R&D activities and provides a list of the sector's current R&D priorities and capability gaps.

7.1 R&D Management Processes

In September of 2007, the HPH Sector formed the JAWG to identify and inform research needs. The JAWG comprises subject matter experts from government and the private sector. Its role is to identify gaps in the sector's ability to prepare for, respond to, and recover from all hazards.

Since its inception, the JAWG has played a significant role in focusing the sector's R&D and MS&A efforts on initiatives that have the greatest potential for reducing the negative consequences of all-hazards events. JAWG members devote significant time and resources to developing R&D and MS&A requirements. The process includes an environmental scan of current and historical research to limit the potential for duplicative projects. The scan occurs at the international level, sector level (e.g., Institute of Medicine, university programs), Federal level (e.g., HHS, DHS S&T Directorate, the National Science Foundation, National Labs, Centers of Excellence), and across the other 17 sectors, particularly those with overlapping functions.

The JAWG reviews its R&D and MS&A portfolio yearly to ascertain how best to allocate time and resources and to review the status of the previous year's efforts. While the JAWG has the primary goal of developing research requirements that are submitted to DHS, the work group also identifies requirements that can be addressed directly by the sector. Such efforts have limited scope and resourcing, but are generally undertaken to address a specific HPH need. The JAWG forms subgroups to lead initiatives that address these needs. Each subgroup has a private sector chair with deep expertise in the research area and a broad constituency from which to draw for additional expertise.

The JAWG develops capability gap statements to describe areas where additional research is needed to improve sector protection and resilience. The JAWG has a vested interest in ensuring that projects that result from the development of capability gap statements progress according to their defined requirements and that, when appropriate, they include sector subject matter experts. JAWG leadership maintains a high degree of visibility into the progress of these projects, reviewing requests for proposals, proposals, and deliverables from each of the initiatives.

The JAWG continuously engages sector partners who are focused on research beneficial to healthcare and public health. Some of the partners include the HHS Agency for Health Research and Quality, Johns Hopkins Preparedness and Catastrophic Event Response (PACER) program, DHS S&T, the National Institute for Hometown Security, the National Biodefense Science Board, the National Infrastructure Simulation and Analysis Center, the Argonne and Pacific Northwest National Labs, and the Institute of Medicine. Through its outreach, the JAWG expands and improves the overall effectiveness of the sector's research and development process.

7.2 R&D Priorities and Capability Gaps

The JAWG has several R&D priorities for the HPH Sector:

- Medical Surge—Enhance the capability to rapidly expand the capacity of the existing healthcare system in response to events.

- Workforce Sustainability—Maintain the HPH workforce during significant events to sustain capacity and reduce impacts to critical functions.

- Medical Supply Chain—Sustain the ability to provide healthcare-related products and services to support critical functions.

- Cyber Infrastructure—Protect HPH cyber systems, networks, and applications.

In 2009, the JAWG submitted 17 capability gap statements in support of these priorities. The gap statements support the sector's four goals of service continuity, workforce protection, physical asset protection, and cybersecurity, and align with the NIPP CIP R&D themes of advanced infrastructure architecture; analysis and decision support systems; entry and access portals; emerging threats and vulnerabilities analysis aides; human and social issues; protection and prevention systems; and response, recovery, and reconstitution tools. Table 7-1 lists the capability gap statements and illustrates their relationship to sector priorities and goals and their alignment with NIPP R&D themes.

Table 7-1: Sector R&D Priorities and Capability Gap Statements Mapped to Sector Goals and NIPP CIP R&D Themes

Priority	Capability Gap Statement	Goals[a]	Themes[b]
Medical Surge	Supply Chain Logistics: Policy and Legal Coordination	SC	AIA, HAS
	Scenario-based Security Assessment Tool	SC, WP, PA	AIA, ADS, RRR
	Cross-Sector Interdependency Analysis	SC	AIA, RRR
	Compound Threat: Cascading Consequence Analysis	SC, WP, PA	AIA, RRR
	Response and Recovery—Long-term Disruptions	SC	AIA, RRR
	Temporary Suspension of Laws to Support Mass Fatalities	SC	HAS
Workforce Sustainability	HPH Workforce Typing	SC	RRR
	Ensuring the Health and Safety of the Nation's Workforce and Families and Dependents	SC, WP	HAS, RRR
	Healthcare Facility Security: Assessing Staff, Patient, and Visitor Perspectives	SC, WP, PA	HAS, PPS
	Assessment and Training of Security Personnel	SC, WP, PA	PPS, RRR
	Identification and Mobilization of an Auxiliary Security Force	SC, PA	HAS, RRR

Priority	Capability Gap Statement	Goals[a]	Themes[b]
Medical Supply Chain	Vulnerabilities in International Supply Chain Manufacturing	SC	AIA, ETV
	Medical Device Sustainability	SC	AIA, RRR
	U.S. Manufacturing Incentives	SC	AIA, PPS, RRR
	Medical Supply Chain: Maintenance of Stockpiles	SC	AIA, RRR
Cyber Infrastructure	Cyber Disruptions to Healthcare and Public Health	SC, CS	AIA, RRR
	Cyber Interdependencies: Cascading Consequences	SC, CS	AIA, RRR

[a] Goal abbreviations: service continuity (SC), workforce protection (WP), physical asset protection (PA), and cybersecurity (CS).

[b] NIPP CIP R&D theme abbreviations: advanced infrastructure architecture (AIA), analysis and decision support systems (ADS), entry and access portals (EAP), emerging threats and vulnerabilities analysis aides (ETV), human and social issues (HSI), protection and prevention systems (PPS), and response, recovery, and reconstitution tools (RRR).

7.3 Path Forward

The HPH Sector has been very successful in building its R&D program through the JAWG and will continue to use this approach. Over the next few years, the focus of the JAWG will shift from the development of new capability gap statements to the implementation and monitoring of research projects that address previously submitted capability gap statements.

Implementation Steps: Research and Development

As in other aspects of healthcare and public health, certain infrastructure protection questions cannot be answered based on current knowledge. HPH Sector organizations can learn more about how to protect their critical assets, systems, and networks by engaging in research and development activities. These are the steps to implement R&D programs:

- Identify knowledge gaps that need to be overcome to meet protection goals.

- Identify partners to assist with research and development.

For additional implementation considerations related to these steps, please see appendix 5.

8. Managing and Coordinating SSA Responsibilities

This chapter describes the management processes and partnership model that HHS uses to meet its responsibilities under HSPD-7 and related guidance. It also describes the information-sharing mechanisms in use in the sector. The chapter provides a path forward for implementing sector partnerships and expanding information sharing in the sector. It also provides a summarized list of implementation actions taken from throughout this plan.

8.1 Program Management Approach

In accordance with HSPD-7, HHS serves as the SSA for the HPH Sector and is responsible for managing and coordinating protection and resilience activities. The Secretary of HHS has delegated leadership responsibility for HSPD-7 to the ASPR, which serves as the HHS Secretary's principal advisory staff on bioterrorism and other public health emergencies and coordinates interagency activities between HHS and other Federal, State, local, tribal, and territorial entities responsible for emergency preparedness and response (EP&R). ASPR has established the CIP Program Office to manage its HSPD-7 responsibilities. The CIP Program Office is integrated with ASPR's EP&R mission, which enables the program to leverage ASPR's relationships and better collaborate with sector stakeholders to advance infrastructure protection goals. On behalf of HHS, the CIP Program Office manages partnerships with all levels of government and the private sector.

8.2 Processes and Responsibilities

8.2.1 SSP Maintenance and Update

The SSP reflects the sector's goals and priorities. The SSA annually reviews and updates the SSP, as warranted by changes in the sector's protection posture, goals, or priorities. Every three years, the SSA and its partners collaborate to issue a more extensive rewrite of the SSP to reflect changes in the program. To ensure accuracy and to reinforce the partnership nature of this effort, the triennial rewrite of the SSP is coordinated with the SCC and GCC before release.

8.2.2 Resources and Budgets

Given the variety of Federal, State, local, tribal, territorial, and private sector partners that contribute funds and other resources to protect the HPH Sector, neither HHS nor any other entity has full authority over resources and budgets for the entire sector. In the Federal Government, a number of departments and agencies outside of HHS own and operate critical infrastructure and are responsible for protecting it. Some Federal departments and agencies also fund programs that protect private sector assets. In HHS, several of the major operating divisions (e.g., CDC, Centers for Medicare & Medicaid Services) manage CIP-related programs. State, local, tribal, and territorial governments manage their own budgets, as do private sector entities. Because ASPR does not have control over these budgets, it must rely on its influence to channel resources toward CIP activities.

To build its influence, ASPR cultivates relationships across the government and in the private sector. In the Federal Government, ASPR engages its counterparts in other departments and operating divisions in HHS. ASPR's RECs conduct outreach to States and localities. The NIPP partnership model enables ASPR to build relationships with the private sector. Through these relationships, ASPR can raise awareness of the CIP program and suggest ways that CIP can be incorporated in planned or existing programs.

8.2.3 Training and Education

The SSA continuously reaches out to educate and inform members of the sector about the CIP program. These outreach and educational activities include presenting at industry conferences, hosting knowledge-sharing sessions, conducting classified briefings, and providing input to CIP-related courses and curriculum.

The SSA attends and presents at sector industry conferences to inform attendees about the CIP program and to provide subject matter expertise concerning various CIP-related topics. Staff from the CIP Program Office present each year at the NACCHO and ASTHO Preparedness Summit and the annual State Directors of Public Health Preparedness Meeting. Representatives from the CIP Program Office attend several other industry conferences, including the Security Analysis and Risk Management Association conference and the Association for Healthcare Resource and Materials Management conference.

The SSA also hosts meetings that enable experts in the sector to share knowledge with each other about specific CIP-related topics. The Continuity of Operations (COOP) meeting is an example. This full-day session brought together thought leaders from across the sector to discuss a number of COOP topics, including legal challenges, patient issues, and methodologies for improved planning, regional programs, security, and facility design. The sector intends to form communities of practice when there is interest in continuing the dialogue from these sessions.

The SSA assists States and localities with the development of CIP programs in their jurisdictions, at their request. While CIP programs vary by jurisdiction, the SSA can share various common approaches for developing and enhancing CIP programs. The SSA also helps connect State, local, tribal, territorial, or private sector CIP programs with key public and private sector entities.

Periodically, the SSA conducts classified threat briefings for members of the sector that have the appropriate security clearance. The intent of these briefings is to provide awareness and education on viable threats faced by the sector. The SSA collaborates with the HHS Office of Security and Strategic Information and DHS HITRAC in preparing and delivering these briefings. In addition to classified briefings, the SSA conducts unclassified briefings with larger audiences to share information with all sector partners. The SSA is committed to producing redacted versions of limited distribution documents and sharing them with broader audiences.

The SSA regularly collaborates with educational institutions to review and provide input to CIP-related courses and curriculum. The sector works with FEMA and other agencies to develop training programs and provide feedback on courses related to the HPH Sector and CIP. Moving forward, the SSA will focus specifically on training that assists private sector partners in engaging Federal, State, and local CIP programs, and that assists State and local partners in establishing these programs.

8.3 Implementing the Partnership Model

8.3.1 NIPP Coordinating Structures

The NIPP partnership model, illustrated in figure 8-1, is the primary organizational structure for coordinating CIP activities. In applying the model, the SSA is responsible for collaborating with public and private sector partners through its SCC and GCC.

The NIPP partnership model encourages collaboration across all 18 sectors through the Federal Senior Leadership Council; the State, Local, Tribal, and Territorial GCC; regional consortia; and the private sector CIKR Cross-Sector Council.

Figure 8-1: Sector Partnership Model

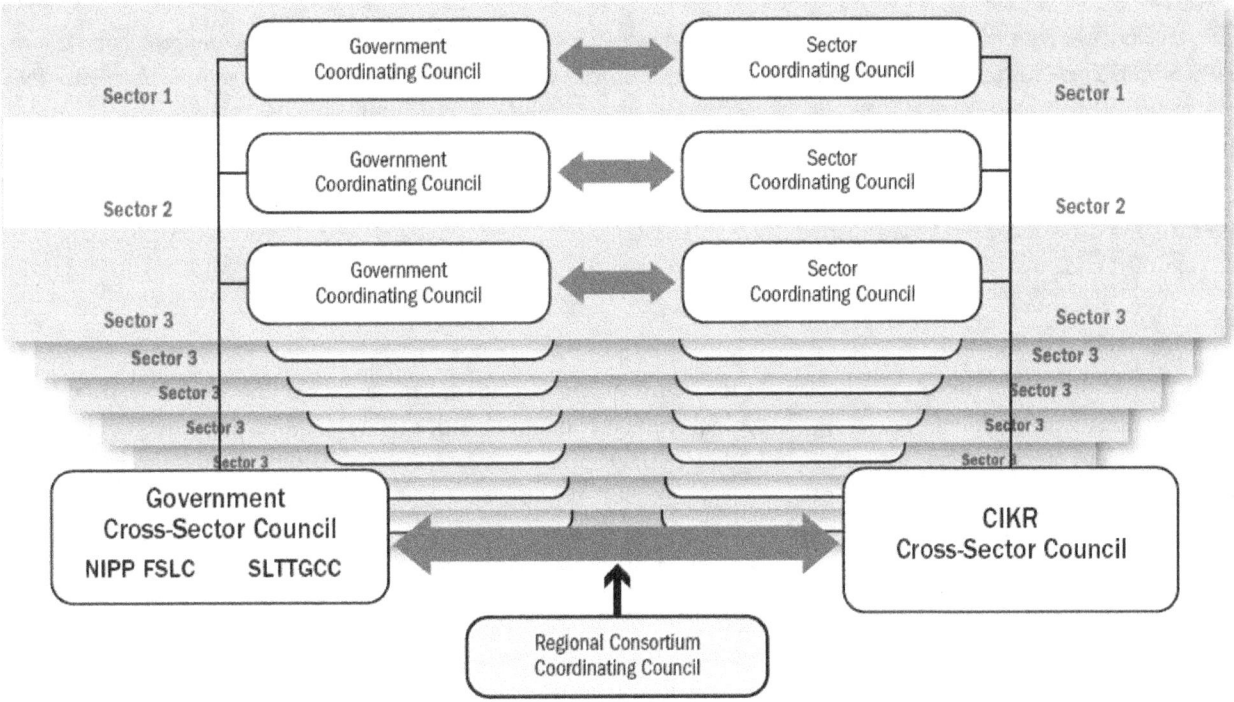

DHS has established the CIPAC to facilitate effective coordination between Federal infrastructure protection programs and the infrastructure protection activities of the private sector and State, local, tribal, and territorial governments. The CIPAC represents a partnership between government and private stakeholders and provides a forum for engaging in a broad spectrum of activities to support and coordinate critical infrastructure protection. CIPAC membership includes representatives from the SCC and GCC. The HPH Sector makes full use of CIPAC to form work groups that carry out its initiatives. This approach has proved very effective in accomplishing sector goals and objectives. Current work groups include the ISWG, JAWG, RAWG, CSWG, and the SAR Writing Work Group.

8.3.2 Advisory Councils and Committees

The HPH Sector participates in several external working groups, including the CSCSWG and the HSPD-21 Biosurveillance Working Group. Through its participation, the sector provides subject matter expertise to the groups and brings back valuable information that informs sector CIP efforts.

The purpose of the CSCSWG is to identify opportunities to improve sector coordination around cybersecurity issues and topics, highlight cyber dependencies and interdependencies, and share government and private sector cybersecurity products and findings. The SSA provides subject matter expertise for development of the National Cyber Incident Response Plan and other work products; reviews the objectives of the working group; and provides relevant feedback to the SCC on cybersecurity initiatives arising from the CSCSWG that affect the sector.

HSPD-21 establishes a National Strategy for Public Health and Medical Preparedness. The Biosurveillance Working Group supports development of this strategy. The SSA participates in the working group to identify sector CIP challenges, inform the direction of the strategy, and improve communication with other working group participants.

8.3.3 Academia, Research Centers, and Think Tanks

The SSA collaborates with various academic institutions and research centers to advance the infrastructure protection efforts of the HPH Sector. These institutions include the Kentucky Critical Infrastructure Program (KY CIP), New York University (NYU), the University of Virginia (UVA), HITRAC, and the Johns Hopkins PACER Center of Excellence.

Through its JAWG, the HPH Sector collaborates closely with academic institutions and research centers. The JAWG partners with KY CIP to fill and contract capability gaps that it has identified. The SSA worked with NYU to conduct a pilot study focusing on theft and diversion. The JAWG is partnering with HITRAC and UVA to provide input to the development of a new risk assessment methodology.

8.3.4 International Organizations

In partnership with the U.S. Department of State, Federal Bureau of Investigation, DoD, and DHS, the SSA maintains relationships with international health organizations, foreign governments, and multinational corporations. The SSA collaborates with international health organizations, including the World Health Organization, Pan American Health Organization, and World Organization for Animal Health to further pandemic preparedness efforts. The SSA also participates in the trilateral Security and Prosperity Partnership Program with Canada and Mexico and coordinates directly with a number of foreign countries on pandemic influenza preparedness and response initiatives. In the private sector, the SSA works with multinational corporations that manufacture medical supplies and equipment outside the United States to manage the risk of supply chain disruption.

8.4 Information Sharing and Protection

The HPH Sector invests significant resources to continually expand its information-sharing capabilities. The sector maintains an active ISWG responsible for overseeing information-sharing initiatives. These initiatives include the enhancement and rollout of the HSIN-HPH portal and the implementation of notification and alert capability. In response to all-hazards events, the SSA initiates conference calls open to the entire sector to accelerate communications. These information-sharing initiatives deliver considerable value to sector members and have significantly increased engagement in the CIP program.

The ISWG is a partnership of government agencies and private sector entities that collaborate to address the information-sharing needs of the sector. The ISWG meets regularly to develop communications and information-sharing strategies for the sector, and to promote information exchange and develop information-sharing procedures.

The HSIN-HPH portal plays a major role in the SSA strategy to facilitate timely and effective sharing of information with sector stakeholders. The main site has general content on CIP in the HPH Sector, while specific subsites are dedicated to ongoing incidents and the many public-private work groups that the sector maintains. The SSA routinely monitors health-related CIP information sources and posts relevant content to the portal. The information covers a broad variety of topics, including policy issues, operations, threat and vulnerability information, and cybersecurity issues. Usage of the HSIN-HPH portal continues to increase at a rapid rate. The SSA coordinates with sector professional and industry associations to distribute invitations to their members describing the value of the portal and providing instructions for requesting an account. This approach has resulted in the addition of hundreds of HSIN-HPH portal account holders.

The SSA makes use of listserv technology to maintain email distribution lists for SCC and GCC members and HSIN-HPH portal users. Sector leadership uses these email distribution lists to notify the sector about CIP-related activities and to send alerts about upcoming meetings on all-hazards events. The HPH Sector is investigating the use of other information-sharing mechanisms to provide urgent alerts to sector members.

To ensure sector partners and stakeholders have timely information about unfolding all-hazards events, the SSA holds regular conference calls with sector members to provide updates and gather pertinent information from owners and operators. The conference calls allow for valuable information exchange that can assist in the response to and recovery from an incident.

Protecting proprietary or sensitive information is essential to the success of information-sharing efforts. The HPH Sector follows a process to ensure that only members of the sector are granted access to the HSIN-HPH portal. The sector posts to the portal only unclassified or For Official Use Only (FOUO) information and follows all formal procedures when holding classified threat briefings.

The SSA is committed to ensuring information sharing at all levels. In addition to maintaining the HSIN portal, the SSA maintains a public CIP Web site, which includes unclassified information available to the general public. The SSA produces FOUO and non-FOUO versions of the SSP and SAR, and will redact classified documents it creates and share them in FOUO format through the HSIN portal.

8.5 The Path Forward

The HPH Sector has been very successful in implementing the partnership model and developing information-sharing capabilities. The sector will continue to make use of the CIPAC framework to establish work groups focused on meeting its goals and objectives. The sector will also continue to expand its use of HSIN-HPH by identifying and posting additional information products and increasing the number of users.

8.6 SSP Implementation Actions

The path forward subsections of this document describe implementation actions that the sector intends to accomplish over the next several years. Table 8-1 provides a summary of these actions.

Table 8-1: SSP Implementation Actions

NIPP Framework Process	Implementation Action
Identify Assets, Systems, Networks, and Functions	Continue defining the functions of the HPH Sector to support an analysis of the underlying infrastructure necessary to perform these functions.
	Increase RAWG involvement in the NCIPP, fully engaging the work group in the information collection and verification processes.
	Develop a more formal list of assets that do not qualify for Level 1/Level 2 designation, but which are still deemed important or critical to the sector.
Assess Risks	Educate the sector on the types and availability of risk assessment tools.
	Leverage network analysis to inform CIP risk mitigation activities.
Prioritize Infrastructure	Continue using NCIPP as the prioritization process, expanding it to include newly identified assets that do not qualify for Level 1/Level 2 designation, but which are still deemed important or critical to the sector.

NIPP Framework Process	Implementation Action
Develop and Implement Protective Programs and Resilience Strategies	Continue to inform senior officials involved in policy development so that their decisions factor in the most critical protection needs of the sector.
Measure Effectiveness	Continue to partner with organizations that fund large CIP programs to leverage their performance management data.
	Work with organizations that fund large CIP programs to add measures to their performance management systems that are CIP-focused.
Continue Research and Development	Continue to use the JAWG as the mechanism for operating the R&D program.
	Shift focus from developing capability gap statements to implementing and monitoring research projects.
Continue Partnership Model	Continue using CIPAC work groups to accomplish sector goals and objectives.
Identify Information-Sharing Products	Identify additional information products to be shared with the sector.
	Continue to increase the number of HSIN-HPH users.

Implementation Steps: Managing and Coordinating Sector-Specific Agency Responsibilities

In many cases, the protection of HPH Sector critical infrastructure will be only one component of a jurisdiction's critical infrastructure protection activities. Any organization involved in HPH Sector infrastructure protection may benefit from coordinating activities and using resources across organizations and jurisdictions. This is the step to manage and coordinate SSA responsibilities:

- Engage in jurisdictional and national critical infrastructure protection efforts.

For additional implementation considerations related to this step, please see appendix 5.

Appendix 1: List of Acronyms and Abbreviations

ASPR	The Office of the Assistant Secretary for Preparedness and Response
ASTHO	Association of State and Territorial Health Officials
BSL	Biosafety Level
CDC	Centers for Disease Control and Prevention
CII	Critical Infrastructure Information
CIKR	Critical Infrastructure and Key Resources
CIPAC	Critical Infrastructure Partnership Advisory Council
COOP	Continuity of Operations
CSCSWG	Cross-Sector Cyber Security Working Group
CSWG	Cyber Security Work Group
DHS	Department of Homeland Security
DoD	Department of Defense
DPHP	Director of Public Health Preparedness
EP&R	Emergency Preparedness and Response
ESF	Emergency Support Function
FDA	Food and Drug Administration
FEMA	Federal Emergency Management Agency
FISMA	Federal Information Security Management Act of 2002
FOIA	Freedom of Information Act
FOUO	For Official Use Only
GCC	Government Coordinating Council
GDP	Gross Domestic Product
HHS	Department of Health and Human Services
HIE	Health Information Exchange
HIPAA	Health Insurance Portability and Accountability Act of 1996

HITRAC	Homeland Infrastructure Threat and Risk Analysis Center
HPH	Healthcare and Public Health
HSA	Homeland Security Advisor
HSIN	Homeland Security Information Network
HSPD	Homeland Security Presidential Directive
IP	Infrastructure Protection
ISWG	Information Sharing Work Group
JAWG	Joint Advisory Work Group for R&D and MS&A
MHS	Military Health System
MS&A	Modeling, Simulation, and Analysis
MSA	Metropolitan Statistical Area
NACCHO	National Association of County and City Health Officials
NCIPP	National Critical Infrastructure Prioritization Program
NIPP	National Infrastructure Protection Plan
PAHPA	Pandemic and All-Hazards Preparedness Act
PBS	Project BioShield
PCII	Protected Critical Infrastructure Information
PIEID	Pandemic Influenza and Emerging Infectious Diseases
PPO	Program Protection Office
R&D	Research and Development
RAWG	Risk Assessment Work Group
REC	Regional Emergency Coordinator
RMA	Risk Mitigation Activity
S&T	Science and Technology
SAR	Sector Annual Report
SCC	Sector Coordinating Council
SHIRA	Strategic Homeland Infrastructure Risk Analysis
SSA	Sector-Specific Agency
SSP	Sector-Specific Plan
VA	Department of Veterans Affairs
VHA	Veterans Health Administration

Appendix 2: Authorities Governing the Sector

This appendix identifies CIP-related Federal, State, and local authorities. The purpose is to summarize the major laws, rules, regulations, executive orders, and other guidance applicable to the protection of sector CIKR.

Federal Authorities

Table A2-1 summarizes the authorities of Federal agencies playing a role in the HPH Sector, grouped by function. Some authorities repeat because they are related to more than one function.

Table A2-1: Summary of Major HPH Sector Federal Authorities by Agency and Function

Types of Authorities	Laws, Regulations, Executive Orders, and Other Authorities
Authorities of Sector-Specific Agencies	
HHS	• Public Health Service Act of 1944 (42 United States Code (U.S.C.) 201-300hh-11), as amended; • Social Security Act of 1935 (42 U.S.C. 1320b-5), as amended; • Federal Food, Drug, and Cosmetic Act of 1938 (21 U.S.C. 301, et seq.), as amended; • Public Health Threats and Emergencies Act of 2000 (Title I of the Public Health Improvement Act (Public Law 106-505)); • Executive Order 13228 establishing the Homeland Security Council, including the Medical and Public Health Preparedness Policy Coordinating Committee; • HSPD-7 18(b) designating HHS as the SSA for healthcare, public health, and food (other than meat, poultry, and egg products), December 17, 2003; and • National Infrastructure Protection Plan, 2009.

Types of Authorities	Laws, Regulations, Executive Orders, and Other Authorities
Authorities Related to Critical Infrastructure Protection	
Responding to All-Hazards	• HSPD-21 establishes a National Strategy for Public Health and Medical Preparedness, October 17, 2007; • Pandemic and All-Hazards Preparedness Act of 2006 (Public Law 109-417); • Department of Defense Instruction (DoDI) 6055.17 "DoD Installation Emergency Management Program" (January 13, 2009); • Intelligence Reform and Terrorism Prevention Act of 2004 (Public Law 108-458); • National Response Framework, 2008; • Emergency Support Function #8, Health and Medical Services Annex, January, 2003; • Public Health Security and Bioterrorism Preparedness and Response Act of 2002 (Public Law 107-188); • Title VIII, Section 817, of the USA Patriot Act of 2001 (Public Law 107-56); • Department of Veteran Affairs Emergency Preparedness Act of 2002 (Public Law 107-287); • Project BioShield Act of 2004 (Public Law 108-276); • Veterans Affairs Department and Department of Defense Health Resources Sharing and Emergency Operations Act of 2002 (Public Law 97-174); • Defense Against Weapons of Mass Destruction Act of 1996 (50 U.S.C. 40); • Public Health Service Act of 1944 (42 U.S.C. 201-300hh-11), as amended; and • Food, Drug, and Cosmetic Act of 1938 (21 U.S.C. 301, et seq.), as amended.
Ensuring Cybersecurity	• HSPD-23: (CLASSIFIED) Computer Network Monitoring and Cyber-Security; • Critical Infrastructure Protection Act of 2001 (Title III, Section 1016, of the USA Patriot Act); • Computer Fraud and Abuse Act of 1984 (18 U.S.C. 1030); • Communications Lines, Stations, or Systems Act of 2002 (18 U.S.C. 1362); • Computer Fraud and Abuse Act of 1984 (18 U.S.C. 1030), as amended by the Computer Abuse Amendments Act of 1994; • Presidential Decision Directive 75 (PDD-75) establishing a counterintelligence role in identifying and protecting critical national assets.
Promoting Information Sharing	• Intelligence Reform and Terrorism Prevention Act of 2004 (Public Law 108-458); • Homeland Security Information Sharing Act (Public Law 107-296), enacted as part of the Homeland Security Act of 2002; • Executive Order 13311 declaring the President's intent to promote information sharing; • Public Health Service Act of 1944 (42 U.S.C. 201-300hh-11), as amended; • Social Security Act of 1935 (42 U.S.C. 1320b-5), as amended; and • Federal Food, Drug, and Cosmetic Act of 1938 (21 U.S.C. 301, et seq.), as amended.

Types of Authorities	Laws, Regulations, Executive Orders, and Other Authorities
Protecting Information	• Critical Infrastructure Information Act of 2002 (Title II, Subtitle B, of the Homeland Security Act); • Electronic Communications Privacy Act of 1986 (18 U.S.C. 2510); • Cyber Security Enhancement Act of 2002 (Title II, Section 225, of the Homeland Security Act of 2002); • Federal Information Security Management Act (Public Law 107-347), Title III of the E-Government Act of 2002; • Health Insurance Portability and Accountability Act of 1996 (Public Law 104-191); • DHS Procedures for Handling Critical Infrastructure Information, Final Rule, 6 CFR Part 29 (September 1, 2006); • Freedom of Information Act and Privacy Act Procedures, DHS Interim Final Rule, (January 27, 2003); • Executive Order 13231, as amended by EO 13286 (dealing with critical information protection); • HHS Standards for Privacy of Individually Identifiable Health Information Regulation Text; Security Standards for the Protection of Electronic Protected Health Information; General Administrative Requirements, including Civil Money Penalties; Procedures for Investigations, Imposition of Penalties, and Hearings (45 CFR Parts 160 and 164), December 28, 2000, as amended (May 31, 2002; August 14, 2003; February 20, 2003; and April 17, 2003); • Economic Espionage Act of 1996 (18 U.S.C. 1831); and • Government Performance and Results Act of 1993 (31 U.S.C. 1115).
Developing and Promulgating Plans	• HSPD-10: Biodefense for the 21st Century. Provides a comprehensive framework for our Nation's biodefense; • Intelligence Reform and Terrorism Prevention Act of 2004 (Public Law 108-458); • Comprehensive Environmental Response, Compensation, and Liability Act of 1980; • Clean Water Act of 1980; • Energy Reorganization Act of 1974; • Project BioShield Act of 2004; • HSPD-3 directing industries to develop their own protective measures (March 11, 2002); • HSPD-7 directing the creation of various infrastructure protection plans (December 17, 2003); • HSPD-8 encouraging greater preparedness on the part of State and local entities against terrorist attacks (December 2003); • PDD-75 establishing a counterintelligence role in identifying and protecting critical national assets; • HHS Continuity of Operations Plan (COOP) for Public Health and Medical Emergencies; • DoD, Strategy for Homeland Defense and Civil Support, June 2005; • DoDI 6200.03 "Public Health Emergency Management Within the Department of Defense" (January 14, 2010); • Public Health Service Act of 1944 (42 U.S.C. 201-300hh-11), as amended; • Social Security Act of 1935 (42 U.S.C. 1320b-5), as amended; • Federal Food, Drug, and Cosmetic Act of 1938 (21 U.S.C. 301, et seq.), as amended; • Executive Order 13347, Individuals With Disabilities in Emergency Preparedness (July 2004); and • The Older Americans Act of 1965 (Public Law 106-501), as amended.

Types of Authorities	Laws, Regulations, Executive Orders, and Other Authorities
Protecting Critical Infrastructure	• The Intelligence Reform and Terrorism Prevention Act of 2004 (Public Law 108-458); • National Strategy for Homeland Security (2007); • National Strategy for the Physical Protection of Critical Infrastructures and Key Assets (2003); • National Response Framework (2008); • Department of Homeland Security Strategic Plan (2004); • Department of Defense Directive (DoDD) 3020.40 "DoD Policy and Responsibilities for Critical Infrastructure" (January 14, 2010); • DoDI 3020.45 "Defense Critical Infrastructure Program Management" (April 21, 2008); • Strategic Plan to Combat Bioterrorism and Other Public Health Threats and Emergencies (2003); • National Infrastructure Protection Plan (2009); and • National Strategy to Secure Cyberspace (2004).
Conducting R&D	• National Science and Technology Policy, Organization and Priorities Act of 1976 (Public Law 94-282); • Title VIII, Section 815, of the USA Patriot Act (October 2001); • Cyber Security Research and Development Act of 2002 (Public Law 107-305); • Project BioShield Act of 2004; • National Plan for Research and Development in Support of Critical Infrastructure Protection of 2004; • Public Health Service Act (42 U.S.C. 201-300hh-11); • Social Security Act of 1935 (42 U.S.C. 1320b-5); and • Federal Food, Drug, and Cosmetic Act (21 U.S.C. 301, et seq.)
Providing Federal Assistance to State and Local Authorities	• Public Health Threats and Emergencies Act of 2000 (Public Law 106-505); • Robert T. Stafford Disaster Relief and Emergency Assistance Act of 2005 (42 U.S.C. 5121 et seq.); • Public Health Service Act (42 U.S.C. 201-300hh-11); • Social Security Act of 1935 (42 U.S.C. 1320b-5); • Federal Food, Drug, and Cosmetic Act (21 U.S.C. 301, et seq.); • DoDD 3025.1, "Military Support to Civil Authorities (MSCA)" (January 15, 1993; and • National Response Framework (formerly the National Response Plan).
Protecting Freedom and Privacy	• Freedom of Information Act of 1966 (5 U.S.C. 552), as amended; • Privacy Act of 1974 (5 U.S.C. 552(a)); • Financial Management Act of 1999 (Gramm-Leach-Bliley); • Government Performance and Results Act of 1993 (31 U.S.C. 1115); and • Standards for Privacy of Individually Identifiable Health Information, Final Rule (42 CFR Part 2).
Protecting Workforces	• The Occupational Safety and Health Act of 1970 (Public Law 91-596), in particular, Section 13, Procedures to Counteract Imminent Dangers; and • Executive Order 13347, Individuals with Disabilities in Emergency Preparedness (July 2004).

State and Local Authorities

Most public health authority is based in the States, typically as an exercise of their police powers.[14] States use this authority in a number of ways to protect public health, including enforcing safety and sanitation codes, conducting inspections, mandating the reporting of certain diseases to State authorities, compelling isolation or quarantine, and licensing healthcare workers

[14] The term "police powers" is derived from the Tenth Amendment to the Constitution of the United States, which reserves to the States those rights and powers not delegated to the U.S. Government. Historically, these have been interpreted to include authority over the welfare, safety, health, and morals of the public.

and facilities. Most States can declare public health emergencies, temporarily expanding their powers still further. States often delegate responsibility for some public health activities to local governments.

Many public hospitals are owned and operated by special districts and governed by their own locally elected officials, who report to their own constituencies. These local governing bodies that own and operate hospitals are not Federal, State, or county agencies. Many have their own ordinance-making authority.

Appendix 3: Healthcare and Public Health Sector Coordinating Council Member Organizations

Abbott

AdvaMed

Aetna

American Academy of Nurse Practitioners

American Academy of Pediatrics

American Academy of Physician Assistants

American Association of Blood Banks

American Association of Colleges of Pharmacy

American Association of Occupational Health Nurses

American Association of Tissue Banks

American College of Emergency Physicians

American College of Occupational and Environmental Medicine

American College of Physicians

American Health Care Association

American Hospital Association

American Industrial Hygiene Association

American Medical Depot

American Nurses Association

American Osteopathic Association

American Red Cross

American Society of Health System Pharmacists

America's Health Insurance Plans

Amgen

Association for Healthcare Resource and Materials Management

Baxter Healthcare

Biotechnology Industry Organization

Blood Centers of America

Blue Cross Blue Shield Florida

Blue Shield California

Blu-Med Response Systems

Brooklawn Memorial Park

Business Continuity Consulting

Cardinal Health

Casket and Funeral Supply Association of America

Catholic Cemeteries, Diocese of Wilmington

Catholic Cemetery Conference

Cisco Systems

Control Risks

Corporate Safety, Security, and Building Services

Cremation Association of North America

Dartmouth Hitchcock Medical Center

Dodge Company

Generic Pharmaceutical Association

Genzyme Corporation

Greater New York Hospital Association

Group Health Cooperative

Gunderson Lutheran Health Plan

Hanover Hospital

Health Industry Distributors Association

Healthcare Distribution Management Association

Healthcare Information and Management Systems Society

Henry Schein

Hospital Association of Southern California

Humana

Independence Blue Cross

International Association for Healthcare Security and Safety

International Cemetery, Cremation and Funeral Association

James B. Haggin Memorial Hospital

Johns Hopkins University

Joint Commission

Kaiser Permanente

Kent and O'Connor

LabCorp

Matthews Cremation

Medline Industries

Memorial Sloan Kettering Cancer Center

MVP Health Care

National Association of Chain Drug Stores

National Association of Nuclear Pharmacies

National Association of Psychiatric Health Systems

National Community Pharmacists Association

National Council of State Boards of Nursing

National Funeral Directors and Morticians Association

Nevada Hospital Association

New England Center for Emergency Preparedness

Operation PAR

Owens & Minor

Pharmaceutical Research and Manufacturers of America

Regence Group

Regional Medical Center

Samaritan Health Services

Hunter College School of Nursing

Siemens Healthcare USA

Terumo Medical Corporation

Texas A&M University

Tuomey Healthcare System

Universal Hospital Services

University of Montana

University of Pittsburgh Medical Center

Walt Disney Company

Washington Occupational Health Associates

WellPoint

Westchester Medical Association

Appendix 4: Healthcare and Public Health Sector Government Coordinating Council Member Organizations

Department of Health and Human Services

- Office of the Secretary
  - Assistant Secretary for Preparedness and Response
  - Assistant Secretary for Health
  - National Coordinator for Health Information Technology
- Operating Divisions
  - Agency for Healthcare Research and Quality
  - Centers for Disease Control and Prevention
  - Centers for Medicare and Medicaid Services
  - Food and Drug Administration
  - National Institutes of Health

Association of Public Health Laboratories

Association of State and Territorial Health Officials

Department of Agriculture

Department of Defense

Department of Energy

Department of Homeland Security

Department of Interior

Department of Labor

Department of Veterans Affairs

Michigan Department of Community Health

National Association of County and City Health Officials

Nassau County Department of Health

Appendix 5: Implementation Considerations for State, Local, Tribal, Territorial, and Private Sector Partners

This appendix provides suggestions and questions that States, localities, tribes, Territories, and private sector partners should consider when establishing their own CIP programs. Considerations are provided for each major chapter of the SSP.

1. Sector Profile and Goals

- Research and describe the HPH Sector in your jurisdiction:
  - What data sources are available on the HPH Sector in my jurisdiction and how can they be accessed?;
  - What are the key public and private sector entities providing healthcare and public health in my jurisdiction?;
  - What impact does healthcare and public health have on my jurisdiction's economy?; and
  - What portion of my jurisdiction's workforce is in the HPH Sector?
- Identify CIP partners:
  - What entity coordinates overall CIP in my jurisdiction and who coordinates it for the HPH Sector? (e.g., HSA, Department of Emergency Management, Health Department);
  - What healthcare and public health associations can be partnered with in my jurisdiction (e.g., State Hospital Association, State Medical Society, State Association of County and City Health Officials, Chamber of Commerce); and
  - What agencies, associations, and companies can be partnered with to address key interdependencies?:
    - Transportation;
    - Communications;
    - Energy;
    - Water;
    - Emergency Services;
    - Information Technology;
    - Postal and Shipping;
    - Chemical; and
    - Food and Agriculture.
- Develop a plan for critical infrastructure protection:

- Does my jurisdiction have a CIP Plan that can guide my planning efforts?;

- What are my entity's CIP goals and objectives? What level of protection can reasonably be provided given local conditions and resources?; and

- What incentives can be identified for private sector participation and how should they be communicated?

2. Identify Assets, Systems, and Networks

- Identify healthcare and public health critical infrastructure for your entity or jurisdiction:

  - Are there assets and systems, whether physical or virtual, so vital that the incapacity or destruction of such may have a debilitating impact on the security, economy, public health or safety, environment, or any combination of these in my jurisdiction?; and

  - What consistent criteria or process would I use to identify such assets?

- Take a broad approach in identifying critical assets and systems:

  - Beyond the most obvious assets (e.g., large hospitals), have I identified key supporting infrastructure?;

  - Have I considered infrastructure that could have a national impact, even though it does not have an immediate State or local impact (e.g., manufacturing and supply chain infrastructure)?; and

  - Has my approach covered all subsectors?:

    - Insurers and payers;

    - Pharmaceuticals, laboratories, and blood;

    - Medical materials;

    - Health information technology; and

    - Mortuary care.

- Become involved in national or jurisdictional data call for CIKR:

  - Is there a State or jurisdictional data call for CIKR? If so, what entity coordinates it?; and

  - Have I identified nationally critical infrastructure that can be reported for the national data call through the State HSA?

3. Assess Risks

- Conduct a hazard vulnerability assessment:

  - Have other entities already conducted assessments that would be useful to me (i.e., HSA, Emergency Management Agency, Health Department)?; and

  - What assessment tools are available to me on the HSIN?

- Match risks against protection goals and objectives:

  - Have I identified risks in the following areas?:

    - Service continuity;

    - Workforce protection;

    - Physical asset protection; and

    - Cybersecurity.

4. Prioritize Infrastructure

- Prioritize hazards and critical infrastructure based on probability and consequence:
  - What prioritization tools are available to me? Are there tools on the HSIN?;
  - What subject matter experts and other partners are available to assist with this process?;
  - What are the highest priority hazards I face?;
  - What infrastructure assets or systems merit the highest protection priority based on risks and consequences?; and
  - How will I verify or validate these priorities?

5. Develop and Implement Protective Programs and Resilience Strategies

- Identify initiatives that are already underway:
  - What government programs are being implemented?; and
  - What voluntary initiatives are private sector partners taking?
- Identify protection gaps:
  - What protection goals and objectives are not addressed by current protective programs?; and
  - Would additional protective programs be helpful?
- Develop risk mitigation activities:
  - What low-cost, voluntary activities might be implemented with the support of private sector partners?;
  - What resources (e.g., Federal and State grants) may be available to implement additional activities?; and
  - In what ways can information sharing be used as a mitigation activity?

6. Measure Effectiveness

- Identify measures of critical infrastructure protection:
  - How can each of the protection goals and objectives be measured?; and
  - How can the sector's participation in CIP activities be measured?
- Identify data sources for measurement:
  - Are there existing grant program reporting requirements that can be used for metrics data?; and
  - What data sources currently exist or are easily obtainable from private sector partners?

7. CIKR Protection Research and Development

- Identify knowledge gaps that need to be overcome to meet protection goals:
  - Are there any components of healthcare and public health delivery in my jurisdiction that are not fully understood?; and
  - Are there any interdependencies in my jurisdiction that are not fully understood?
- Identify partners to assist with research and development:
  - Are there State or local universities or associations that can provide assistance?; and
  - Are there research and development activities at the Federal level that might assist me?

8. Managing and Coordinating Sector-Specific Agency Responsibilities

- Engage in jurisdictional and national CIP efforts:

  - Have we reached out to our jurisdictional partners for critical infrastructure protection?;

  - Have I registered for the HSIN portal for healthcare and public health?; and

  - Are the national associations that represent me or my entity engaged in national CIP efforts? Have I discussed these issues with the association?

Please direct any questions or comments to **cip@hhs.gov**